Praise for *True Secrets of Lesbian Desire*
(*Love's Learning Place,* in hardcover):

"Renate Stendhal shows us, reassuringly and lovingly, how cultivating radical honesty — about who we are, where we've been, what we want, and how we want it — gives us the tools to start creating the relationships and sex lives we really want, without starting over from scratch."

    — Hanne Blank, author of *Big Big Love: A Sourcebook on Sex for People of Size and Those Who Love Them*

"This lovely book offers sound advice on how to relate with one's lover. Its emotionally honest tone posits that trust and truth are keys to unlocking long-term erotic pleasure. Stendhal is playful, practical, and philosophical. She is a warm teacher whose wisdom belongs in the life of every lesbian stuck on the myth of lesbian bed death."

    — Richard Labonte, *BookMarks, Q-Syndicate*

"A few self-help books tackle women's issues with a more politicized lens and increased sensitivity. *True Secrets* examines women's long-term relationships and asserts that truth telling as political act can create a deeper love and is the healthiest, 'least costly,' and most effective strategy available."

    — Nicole Braun, *Foreword*

"Stendhal is onto something. *True Secrets* is the start of serious dialogue on lesbian relationships, emphasizing their validity and showing that, like any other relationship, they are worth working for."

    — Jano, *Lambda Book Report*

"This book is a welcome addition to the small number of lesbian self-help psychology books on the market. Using examples of couple interaction in therapy sessions, Stendhal cites cases from her practice in which self-awareness was achieved. She takes special aim at the shame some women experience around sex."

    — Sonja Franeta, *The Gay and Lesbian Review*

BOOKS BY
RENATE STENDHAL

Sex and Other Sacred Games
(with Kim Chernin)

Gertrude Stein in Words and Pictures

Cecilia Bartoli: The Passion of Song
(with Kim Chernin)

The Grasshopper's Secret

True Secrets
of Lesbian Desire

Keeping Sex Alive
in Long-Term Relationships

RENATE STENDHAL

North Atlantic Books
Berkeley, California

Published by:

North Atlantic Books   Cover Design by Jan Camp
P.O. Box 12327   Cover Image by Eric Boutilier-Brown
Berkeley, California 94712

Printed in the United States of America

First published in the United States by Edgework Books as *Love's Learning Place: Truth as Aphrodisiac in Women's Long Term Relationships*.

True Secrets of Lesbian Desire is sponsored by the Society for the Study of Native Arts and Sciences, a nonprofit educational corporation whose goals are to develop an educational and crosscultural perspective linking various scientific, social, and artistic fields; to nurture a holistic view of the arts, sciences, humanities, and healing; and to publish and distribute literature on the relationship of mind, body, and nature.

North Atlantic Books' publications are available through most bookstores. For further information, call 800-337-2665 or visit our website at www.northatlanticbooks.com.

Substantial discounts on bulk quantities are available to corporations, professional associations, and other organizations. For details and discount information, contact our special sales department.

Library of Congress Cataloging-in-Publication Data

Stendhal, Renate, 1944–
    True secrets of lesbian desire : keeping sex alive in long-term relationships / by Renate Stendhal.
    p. cm.
Includes bibliographical references.
    ISBN 1-55643-475-8
    1. Sex instruction for lesbians. 2. Lesbians—Sexual behavior.
3. Lesbians—Attitudes. 4. Lesbians—Psychology. 5. Intimacy (Psychology) I. Title.
    HQ75.51.S74 2003
    306.76'63—dc22

                                                    2003005463
                                                    CIP

    1 2 3 4 5 6 7 8 9 DATA 07 06 05 04 03

Every part of you has a secret language.
Your hands and your feet say what you've done.
And every need brings in what's needed.
Pain bears its cure like a child.
Having nothing produces provisions.
Ask a difficult question,
And the marvelous answer appears.

— Rumi

Table of Contents

FOREWORD

The crude and inaccurate messages we receive from the culture are all white noise, drowning out the many truths about who we are and where our desire lies. They are the old stories; they make us afraid. The longer we're in a relationship the louder the noise gets. The rituals of regularity, the comfort of familiarity, the satisfaction of finding our mate, and the excitement of sex can all lead us, paradoxically, away from intimacy and truth-telling. It's as if the driver on the wonderful road trip becomes preoccupied with the signs for exits to Motel 6 and WalMart. On the way we see nothing but the signs, while the true landscape is obscured.

Using the paradigm of the therapeutic setting and examining the "noise" around us, Renate Stendhal in *True Secrets of Lesbian Desire* points to the paths that lead to healthy sexual lives within the framework of the relationships we've chosen. By focusing on three sets of couples she teaches in the "truth-telling" she advocates, Stendhal shows how the paralyzing fear of revealing ourselves to our beloved can be seen as a wall right down the middle of the bedroom. Because we are women, we've been taught to vacuum around the impediment and not mention it out loud, even when it concerns our own sexual pleasure. Chipping down the wall between ourselves and a lover is as full-time a job as any nine-to-five. This learning and relearning require commitment much stronger than any matrimonial ceremony can guarantee.

Stendhal examines the "shadow" in lesbian relationships that descends when women bond so completely that the intimacy becomes a merging, obliterating the space between individuals

where desire lies. Lesbian bed death, the topic of so many comediennes, is examined and reined in, no longer an inevitable result of a solid relationship.

True Secrets casts an eye on the myths that burden us all. Stories larger than our lives make promises to us about how we will love and desire. These are myths we can learn to see past when we analyze them head-on. As we make our own paths through the muck and mire, we create a sense of both safety and excitement, one of the most important combinations any of us can hope to achieve in a relationship.

We unwittingly embrace isolation, cloaked in such phrases as "It's too scary to share that with her," or "This feeling makes me look like a fool," or "She has more experience than I do — she should be able to solve this!" or "We're both women, she should know what I want." The phrases have endless variations, but the final result is to separate you from your deepest desires and from the one who might share them. And whether we are looking for love from another woman at 20 or 50 or 200, like my character Gilda, the fears are the same.

Renate Stendhal can help us make our way on roads where we must learn to read the signs *and* look at the scenery. The heated moment between us when ecstasy and affection flame up is often fleeting, but can carry us through decades of days. In her exuberant, joyful, and positive style, Stendhal is a sure driver and guide. Listen in as she shares what she's learned and has taught so many couples for the past few decades.

—Jewelle Gomez
San Francisco, California

Preface to the Second Edition

This second edition of Love's Learning Place is called *True Secrets of Lesbian Desire*. I want to tell you about the beauty and hopefulness lovers find when they begin telling each other their erotic truth. It's easy to say: "Couples need to communicate better! Sex is communication!" The language of intimate, passionate communication has to be invented and learned with every lover. The subtle truth of the body and its sensations tends to come in the form of revelations and confessions about the disappointment and resentment we feel about what our lover does or does not do. It comes as whispered secrets about what we wish to do to our lover, or long for our lover to do to us. When lovers master this language and refine the art of listening to the body, committed monogamy does not lead to sex-starved boredom. On the contrary. I claim that it is precisely in long-term relationships that growing intimacy can nourish sexual passion.

In *True Secrets of Lesbian Desire* we meet three couples, Lou and Annie, Sybil and Mariushka, Petra and Selena. We hear about their different sexual frustrations and watch them enter what I call "love's learning place" where they begin to listen and find words for intimate secrets they never dared to tell each other. On this path of discovering and teaching each other the alphabet of their bodies, their passion is rekindled in surprising ways. All three couples fall in love again or, in my words, "ripen into love." They discover that with enough truth-making there is more than enough love-making.

When I give talks as a counselor for lesbian couples, women often want to know my own true secret: was I ever a victim of bed death? The answer is yes. In my youth I considered bed death inevitable in a long-term relationship. Monogamy seemed a sure-fire condemnation to sexual boredom. I wrestled with the beast all through my feminist-activist years in Europe, with my lovers, and in my writing. Experience taught me that desire was doomed to die a slow death, but intuition told me otherwise. There had to be a way to reconcile lasting love and hot sex.

There are periods in human life when monogamy seems too hard to manage — when it is too much of a struggle against our hormones, or a contradiction to the mood of a time. Such a time for me was during the second wave of feminism in the seventies. In Paris, where I lived, the political and consciousness-raising groups, action committees and assemblies saw a daily stream of new women pouring in — every one of them a potential seductress or object of desire. Entire countries were swept by a woman-identified, woman-loving, lesbian euphoria. The erotic capacities of women seemed limitless: woman with two, three, a whole collective, a roomful of women. Obviously, in this high tide of sexual celebration, monogamy didn't stand a chance.

During my years of multiple relationships, I rarely admitted to myself that something was amiss. My adventures, affairs and "polyamorous" experiments turned out to be emotionally or intellectually frustrating and bogged down in jealousy and deceit. Sexual excitement was short-lived. Was I still searching

for "the right woman?" Was that a romantic myth? I became convinced that the forever sexually attractive, interesting, and engaging woman of my dreams did not exist.

When I seriously fell in love again, at the age of forty-one, I was surprised and — in spite of my delight — suspicious. I moved to Berkeley, California, in the mid-eighties to be with this woman, who was also a writer and feminist, who loved French culture and German poetry. But I was determined not to stay a day longer than my sexual passion lasted.

Seventeen years later, my early intuition has been confirmed: passion and intimacy don't exclude each other. Lasting desire is possible in a relationship if the lovers are compatible, share important interests, like each other in a way best friends do, remain attracted to and curious about each other, and, most importantly, are able to risk honesty with each other.

I have become convinced that truthfulness about feelings and body sensations is the key to lasting passion. Most relationship counselors and sex educators agree about the value of honesty in any ethical, moral, loving relationship. But who ever thought that honesty could be erotic? That truth could be an aphrodisiac? Now I know that it is possible to keep love and sex alive over the years... and perhaps forever, until death do us part.

—Renate Stendhal
Berkeley, California
September 2003

I

A Woman Appeared

Ultimately we know deeply that the
other side of every fear is a freedom.

— *Marilyn Ferguson*

An Approach

The puzzles of love and sex, sex and truth have always
intrigued me. The first book I published in Berkeley, co-
authored with my partner, Kim Chernin, was *Sex and Other
Sacred Games,* a story about two very different women, a lesbian feminist and a femme fatale, debating a central question:
What happens to desire and sexual attraction in a long-term
relationship? Is monogamous sex doomed to die from boredom? Is closeness an obstacle to desire? Can hot sex and intimacy
ever be compatible? These, I think, are questions many of us
are asking.

In *Sex and Other Sacred Games,* one of the women claims that
two committed partners can keep sex alive if they can keep truth
alive. She says, "Truth, I imagine, is the most powerful aphrodisiac of all." What is she saying, exactly? That there is some
special connection between love, sex, and truth? That truth is a

turn-on? More effective than booze, drugs, pain, or separation?

Before writing *Sex and Other Sacred Games,* I had been in consciousness-raising groups in Paris, was involved in feminist projects all over Europe, had led workshops, and had written and lectured on the topic of women's eros and sexuality. After my move to California, I studied psychology and started working as a therapist. I have since talked about sex with many women in my counseling practice, friendships, and social circles. Sex has been a mystery, a torment, and a passionate quest for me from the time of my first teenage diaries. I would brood over my existing or nonexisting sex life, over the difference between men and women, over the handicap of being part of the "second sex." In the famously dark continent of women's sexuality, I was trying to find my own answers to Freud's question, "What do women want?"

Therefore, *True Secrets of Lesbian Desire* reflects several things: A tradition of feminist thinking; my own experience with both women and men; and what I learned from the couples and singles with whom I talked and worked.

The erotic heroines of this book are Annie and Lou, Sybil and Mariushka, Petra and Selena — three couples who came to talk to me about sex. Too much sex in one case, not enough in another, no sex at all in the third. We will follow the couples in their struggles to address their frustrations and save their relationships, and we will see the role truth plays in it all. Telling the truth is a skill that deserves to be learned and refined. The stories of these couples will show that it can be learned, and that one doesn't have to be a master at it before reaping the erotic benefits.

In addressing an intimate and challenging topic like sex, it is only fair for the author to give her readers a basic idea of where she comes from.

D'où tu parles? This was the ethical motto the French feminist movement established from the get-go for all kinds of communication in groups and assemblies. *D'où tu parles?* — literally, "Where do you speak from?" — meant, *Tell us where you come from, give us a background, a perspective, a tool that allows us to understand what you are going to say. Let's remember that all we know, and therefore all we can say, is personal, is a particular viewpoint based on one woman's experience, her class, race, gender awareness, economic and sexual situation, her thoughts, her politics, her philosophy. Let's not assume that we are speaking for anybody else, or generalize and thereby necessarily leave out a multitude of other, different worlds our sisters have experienced.*

The personal was, indeed, political. This radical demand to remain specific and not bury the differences between women in generalizations went directly against our newly born enthusiasm and the radical need to say "we": We are sisters, we are women, we are one breathtaking power....

I admit that I still like to say "we", and not only because I am weary of "you" language. If I say, for example, "If you have sex with a stranger...," it may sound as though I am excluding myself from such a proposition (which I certainly don't). My saying "we" is not meant as an exclusion of difference, but rather as a welcoming gesture, an offer to acknowledge potential similarities. "We," for me, stands for *many of us, some of us,*

at least *a few of us;* and at the very, very minimum, *at least two.*

My "we" always implies that I am not speaking from the assumption that I know about *you* or know anything better than you know it yourself. You, dear reader, are welcome to include yourself to your heart's content, particularly if you recognize your experience in the ways I ponder certain questions, or in the ways the couples I present are struggling through their sexual challenges. Language is tricky, as we will see many times in these notes, but it always leaves us a choice: A deliberate decision, moment by moment, about whether we would like, want, or wish to include ourselves. This is already the threshold where wanting, or desire, begins.

"Whence Speakest Thou?"

My upbringing was rather puritanical, which was typical for the middle classes in postwar Germany. I remember the first years of my life in Berlin, after the war and the Berlin blockade, when my extended family was hunting for food and other life essentials. My Communist grandfather kept rabbits, ducks, and chicken in our little garden, where he grew his tobacco next to the potatoes. All around, there was a chaotic, adventurous, creative spirit of survival against all odds. By the mid-fifties, however, Germany had resettled into getting rich and respectable. Guilt and shame about the immediate past —the Nazi terror, the massacre of the Jews, the lost war

— had been buried under a leaden blanket of silence. The country (and with it, most families like mine) had thrown itself into the obsessive activities and rewards of the Economic Miracle.

A new moralistic terror reigned: That of "good manners" and cleanliness. Middle-class families could afford to shut themselves up in their own apartments or houses, in the sanctified cage of the nuclear family where father knew best. The education of a girlchild was confined within the corset of sexual ignorance, fear, and shame. There were a few books on sexual education aimed at young adults, and I remember earnest discussions with my mother and girlfriends about "waiting for the right man." I had no idea that there was anything like masturbation for a woman until I was twenty-one, and peeked by chance at the Kinsey Report.

By that time, my intimate relations with men and my un-fulfilled yearnings for women had thrown me into an existential despair. I was part of a small group of mostly male intellectuals and artists who considered me their muse or possible lover, but never their equal. In the dominant male view of that time and this milieu, which I could not yet challenge, a woman was not seriously regarded as a thinker, creator, or artist. (Powerful writers like Gertrude Stein or Virginia Woolf were the exceptions that only prove the rule.) Sexuality, as I experienced it, was consen-sual rape, involving people who were clueless about anything concerning the body and its feelings. My compliance with the dictates of the feminine role was "perfect," as my entire educa-tion as a girlchild intended it to be, bringing me to the edge of suicide. The denial of my truth as a thinking, feeling, sexual human being seemed to mirror the entire country's denial of its own painful truth. I knew I had to get away. If I ever wanted to

think and move and breathe freely, I had to become an exile.

When I settled in Paris, at twenty-three, I met the first (at least to my knowledge) real, live lesbian I had ever encountered. We became friends, and a few years later, confessed our attraction to each other. Literally overnight, my life began to make sense. In this first night of love I came to my senses in every sense of the term. It was the beginning of a long journey out of feminine sexual victimhood and into female sexual agency.

This voyage of awakening to my own body and self was soon shared by the many newly minted feminists gathering in Paris. Everyone suddenly was on a "voyage of women becoming," as the American feminists had taught us to call it. Paris, where I spent almost twenty years, provided the sexual challenges and sexual healing I needed. The city dazzled me as a place where women were comparatively "masculine" and men "feminine," and where sex was mythically romanticized and celebrated — among lesbian-feminists as much as among heterosexuals. The people I sought out were extroverted, uninhibited, playful; the women were astonishing in the agility of their minds, their verbal power, their sexual daring. If I wanted to be part of this glittering, brilliant, romantic world, I had to change from the inside out. Something in me resonated with what I perceived as irresistible freedom, even before the sexual revolution and the feminist movement broke the ground and created new concepts for this all-encompassing liberation.

After many years of directing my own sexual education in Paris, I came to see myself as a "liberated woman," or what some perhaps would call a promiscuous adventurer. There were times when I walked through the streets dressed as a boy, lining up with the men in front of Arabian bordellos to peek into a

courtyard filled with women. In this disguise, I dared go to pornographic movies in the racy Pigalle district. I exchanged amorous glances with gay men in the Metro. I loved this role. I loved being followed by gay men through the streets.

The earliest days of the feminist movement had featured sexual orgies, and my interest in exploring threesomes (or more) remained consistent. Like most of my feminist sisters in Paris, I scorned monogamy. One of my passionate relationships had turned into a thirteen-year friendship, but I was convinced that one woman could never satisfy my needs; that even the best meeting of likes and tastes, temperament and intellect, creative endeavors and artistic visions would end up sexless and boring after about two years. I practiced a rigorous division between mind and body, emotional and sexual needs, convinced that they could never be brought together. Just before I left Paris, I was having a regular affair with an Italian woman whenever we happened to meet up. I had a long-term romantic liaison in Zurich, a dependable erotic friendship in Hamburg, and a postsexual life companion in Copenhagen. A number of us were planning to move to the south of France together to build a community and creative center for women.

Then a woman appeared: An American who laughingly claimed that I would never find life with her boring. I accepted the challenge and set sail for California — another culture and language — and plunged into the risks and perils of serious committed monogamy, in which French feminist culture had not particularly specialized.

As I write this, sixteen years of this relationship have passed. Indeed, it has not been boring. I had to recognize that the

consciousness-raising and emotional engagement needed to maintain a fulfilling monogamous relationship are all-consuming. It took intensive learning about myself and my lover, as well as persistent struggle, to undo my past and its false beliefs and skepticism. Many of my old inhibitions resurfaced now that I faced the risks of sexual intimacy. The same, of course, was true for my lover, and there were times when both of us engaged in serious therapy in order to understand ourselves and what we were going through with each other.

To sum up "where I speak from": I can say that my initial skepticism about monogamy has turned into an optimism mixed with persistent amazement about what is possible between two people who like and love each other, are a match for each other, and are committed to telling each other the truth to the best of their capacity.

Entering

First, a passage from *Women and Honor: Some Notes on Lying,* by Adrienne Rich:

> An honorable human relationship — that is, one in which two people have the right to use the word "love" — is a process, delicate, violent, often terrifying to both persons involved, a process of refining the truths they can tell each other. It is important to do this because it breaks down human self-delusion and isolation. It is important to do this because in so doing we do justice to our own complexity. It is important to do this because we can count on so few people to go that hard way with us.

In this powerful essay, written in 1975, Adrienne Rich focuses on the damaging effects of lying; she is not concerned with the erotic effects of truth-telling. Lies and silence do, indeed, constitute an undertow that erodes relationships. However, when two people make honesty part of their communication, the "delicate, violent, often terrifying process" of refining truth has an impact on body and soul. Breaking down "human self-delusion and isolation," doing "justice to our own complexity," "going that hard way together" has the unexpected physical reward of setting love free. The ensuing heart-to-heart closeness, the mutual gratitude and respect, allow for a tenderness that opens the body's urge to break down barriers and melt into erotic desire.

Tenderness breaking into erotic desire?

With a single leap, we have arrived at the paradox of the infamous "lesbian bed death." Ever since the high tide of feminism in the seventies began to ebb, women's relationships have been

under suspicion: There is supposedly too much tenderness and too much closeness. Women couples, we are told, tend to merge and therefore lose their sexual appetite. I doubt that anything could be that simple.

The term "lesbian bed death" was apparently coined by lesbian comedian Kate Clinton. When I first heard the term, I thought it expressed a good deal of self-irony and humor about the well-known fact that a few years into any committed relationship, sex tends to go AWOL. "Lesbian bed death," to my ears, affirms lesbian reality in a culture that still prefers not to know that there is anything like desire and sex between women. If we can publicly mourn and laugh about the death of sex in this way, we implicitly affirm that desire and sex between women are a fact. For something to die, it must once have been living. It must once have been so strong that we can afford to come out of the closet and speak the truth about its absence. And even joke about it.

But the good joke was quickly coopted and used to ridicule supposedly sexless lesbians. The tired old taunt, "How could anybody do it without a penis?" was conveniently refreshed by some sexual surveys claiming that lesbians had sex less often than heteros, even though other studies proved the contrary. Some of the scorn came from the proud tribe of S/M lesbians who referred to their sisters as "vanilla lesbians" (in contrast, perhaps, to their own hot pepper).

Noting how the term "lesbian bed death" was misunderstood and coopted, a number of feminists now don't consider it politically correct. Psychologist and sex therapist Suzanne Iasenza, for example, tries hard to make people aware that if there is any bed death, then men, women, heteros, homos, bisexuals

— everyone has the same potential to succumb to it.

Are we sufficiently aware?

How do we explain the millions and millions of Viagra pills consumed by the men of our society, unless they are constantly threatened by insufficient desire and difficulty sustaining it? But men don't circulate jokes about "hetero bed death." Lack of sexual desire for a man is a deadly serious matter; a matter of identity.

This brings us to the question of what, in our culture, defines sex. What is sex? We know the countless sexual surveys that ask us, "How often do you have sex?" We are not asked, "How often are you intimately close with your partner? How often do you make love? What does lovemaking consist of for you? How do you define sex in your relationship? Do you consider cuddling, holding, stroking, kissing, or gazing 'sex'?"

One client of mine used to reach the height of orgasmic pleasure with her partner by getting a foot massage — but according to the surveys, she had no sex. For heterosexual men, who generally invent these surveys, nongenital sex doesn't count and therefore is not counted. Sex without penetration is not really sex, as we have learned the easy way, thanks to Bill Clinton.

I would argue that this dominant, narrow view of sex as penetration is precisely what preordains sexual bed death for everyone in our culture, where intimate closeness and sexual desire have been split apart. Lack of sex in intimate long-term relationships therefore is a predicament that we could call, taking off from Freud, "Socialization and Its Discontents." We are discontented because we grow up alienated from our bodies, separated from our feelings and primordial longings.

All of us, to some degree, grow up in fear and terror of sexuality, of the power inherent in it. Most women of my generation (I was born in 1944) share the experience of growing up with the denial of our sexual power and potency, the denial of any sexual agency. We had no say and we did not know how to say no. When we look a little more closely at a tossed-off remark like "We had no say," it becomes apparent that so many of our feminist strivings have been an attempt to give us a voice; to create a language, a concept, a world that would allow women to express ourselves and be heard.

Unspeakable Depth

Even though we have changed the world to some degree, there is a realm where we find ourselves, over and over again, speechless — speechless sometimes with confusion, because the words available for our use seem useless. This is the realm of sex, passion, desire, love. Our culture does not provide a language for differentiated exploration of feelings linked to the body and the powerful emotions engendered by love and sex. In the poor, rudimentary language of this culture, women's bodies and experience hardly exist.

Perhaps you remember or have heard about the profound upset in the feminist community following the eruption of the pornography debate, in the early eighties. In a new preface to her essay, "Compulsory Heterosexuality and Lesbian

Existence," Adrienne Rich sums it up: "There has recently been an intensified debate on female sexuality among feminists and lesbians, with lines often furiously drawn, with sadomasochism and pornography as key words which are variously defined according to who is talking." We are indeed furiously debating something we do not even have language for. We have a patriarchally formed and deformed language for love and sex, a "pornographic language." Sadly, if we are realistic, we have to admit that the feminist dream of remaking language in our own image has not yet come true. To use a well-known example from a different culture: The Inuit language, we are told, has thirty-six words for the color of snow. If it became somehow crucial to us to speak about the specific color of our snow, the English language would not be of much help. What to do with a language that doesn't fit us, doesn't mirror us, doesn't contain us? How to express ourselves and tell our truth? What if the thirty-six colors of erotic desire cannot be perceived unless the thirty-six words are available to choose from?

This is the big one, the question that has been pondered by any woman who has tried to think for herself. Ever since Simone de Beauvoir lifted women's condition as "the second sex" into larger awareness, the question has been debated by feminist writers, philosophers, and linguists — with varying degrees of hope and despair. We only need to pick a word at random, like "masturbation," to experience the discrepancy between this medical-logical, prurient sound and the indescribable delight of giving ourselves pleasure. We only need think of a name or concept like "lesbian" or "lesbian bed death" to enter the labyrinth of complications into which the use or nonuse of a word leads us.

Our paucity of language is particularly painful when it comes to sex and to the truth of feelings. Our first experience of everything concerning the body and its emotions happens before we have any language for it. Language develops between the ages of one and two. But anyone who has observed a child at this age knows the full scale of passions, desires, terrors, rages, joys, and ecstasies this tiny human being has already gone through by the time language arrives. We have experienced the depths of what intimacy is made of — dependence, anguish, safety, need, satisfaction, craving, oneness, and loss — before we have names for any of it. This is precisely what we call "unspeakable depths."

Imagine for a moment how it would be to grow up in a land where a child would be taught an "Inuit language" for all the shades of feelings and body sensations. The caretakers in that village would name for the child the violent joys and pains she has to live through. They would do so with patience, tenderness, consistency. Instead of an adult scowl — "How dare you talk to me like that?!" — the adult would reflect back to the child her right to be angry or upset, enraged or outraged. By embracing her feelings in this way and naming them for her, that adult would give the child permission to feel. With permission to feel come tools and techniques to face and embrace whatever is felt and expressed in the true power of the emotion. By "tools and techniques," I mean an emotional, conceptual, verbal safety net that would keep the child from the terror of being overwhelmed by her feelings to the point of falling apart, disintegrating, splitting. I imagine a girl who would feel safe to be angry, to express her rage.

The same would be true, in this utopian village, of all the other basic human feelings — especially the experiences

of pleasure and desire. Vast permission would be granted for every sensual and sexual stirring in the body, solidly governed by mature women's wisdom of what might be safe for a particular child. The caretakers would watch her go after her stirrings with benevolence and humor, naming for her what these joys and appetites are, and teaching her ways to handle them without getting into serious danger and dangerous hurt.

If we hold this utopian vision next to the childhood experiences we remember or choose not to remember, we have the explanation for much confusion, fear, sadness, and rage about sex. The frowns, the scoldings, the shaming looks, the slaps and beatings, the disapproving gazes, the harsh words, the threats, the cold silences that accompanied self-sexual exploration for many of us of the postwar generation certainly didn't encourage the development of knowledge or language for bodily sensation. Indeed, for some, they may have succeeded in eliminating body experience altogether. For younger generations, there may have been a much more positive party line about sex, but in my work with young and younger women I find that even if they are freer to act than were women of my generation, many heterosexual women still have to contend with a perceived sexual powerlessness and a familiar split between sexual sensation and emotion. Young lesbians today often struggle with a similar free-for-all meaninglessness of sex and with the remnants of the old crushing (self-)judgment for being "queer," or "weird" outlaws, as I have heard them describe themselves.

As Dorothy Allison puts it in her essay "Public Silence, Private Terror":

Grief should not be where we have to start when we talk
of sex. But the idea of a life in which rage, physical fear,

or emotional terror prevents even the impetus of desire — that is the image that haunts the discussion for me. The thought that we could all be forced to live isolated in our own bodies, never safe enough to risk ourselves in naked intimacy with others, rides me like an old nightmare from my childhood....

In order to break out of this isolation, we need to communicate; we need to build words, sentences, a language capable of conveying bits of our truth. We need to connect what our bodies do, what our hands and lips do (or want to do), with these bits of naming. There is a connection between ourselves and our bodies that we need to make with the help of this language we are creating. This language, then, is the building block of our ability to reach, touch, and communicate with another person; to know and speak our most personal and private truth.

This is where the difficulties begin and this is where all hope resides. Every one of us is virgin territory, so to speak. Every word can be remade in our own image, if we have the courage to claim words, make them up, reshape, reinvent them, in our dialogue with our lover. Only two people need know this language, which they have made together. Every new person who comes close to us teaches us new words, learns ours, and melds these two intimate languages into speech. What I am describing here is what of course many couples already know, often however without any awareness that they have their own language. The private language of most couples contains childlike transgressions, endearments, and silliness, together with a private code for sex and the body taboos. Once we become aware of this spontaneous verbal inventiveness in our relationships, we can learn

to use these building blocks to build easier roads and bridges between ourself and our lover — pathways of communication and erotic flow. Then, with this new vocabulary, we can begin to answer the disturbing question of why our culture is so obsessed with sex.

Why, then, is our culture so obsessed with sex? Perhaps we are indeed all part of a desperate quest for reunion with the body. Perhaps we long to take possession of it again, to be reconnected, to inhabit our body the way we once did in the lost paradise of body-childhood, to feel the grounding and blissful balance of being embodied again.

If sex is one way to bring us back into this lost paradise, how can we manage to remain there? And what's truth got to do with it?

In this book, we will leave the narrow constraints of what sex is supposed to be, and see a whole new territory open up. Sex is the undiscovered continent of feeling and sensation that can be entered by two people who have made erotic truth part of their commitment. The path I have in mind is difficult but rewarding. In the tender and bold unveiling of intimate body-truth, closeness and sex reveal themselves as compatible.

In *True Secrets of Lesbian Desire* we go beyond the well-known alphabet of the Archetypal Passion with its pining and forbidden fantasies, its longing for the distant, ever-elusive lover, the dangerous, irresistible stranger — stereotypical fantasies that burn up and die as soon as we become intimate. Instead, we learn our uniquely personal alphabet of how to find, invent, give, and receive body-pleasure. We discover the aphrodisiac of truth, and begin to spell out a new erotic language of intimacy that can be spoken until we die.

II

The Thirty-Six Colors

of Erotic Desire

Perhaps everything terrible in us is in its deepest
being something helpless that needs help.

— *Rainer Maria Rilke*

Getting Down To It

Lou and Annie are in their early fifties and have been together for nine years. Lou has a salt-and-pepper crew cut,
Annie a blond bob. They come to sessions in jeans and de-
signer sweatshirts. Lou and Annie have remodeled their house
together and built up a successful desktop publishing business. Over the years, tensions have been building around the
absence of sex from their life as a couple. They present their
problem in the first session.

"We have such a great relationship!" Annie shakes her head
in disbelief. "I mean, we agree about most things, we are both
totally involved in our business, we have almost the same golf
handicap. We love our life together. So why don't we have a
sex life any more? I am only fifty-one, and that's too young to

give up on sex, if you ask me!"

She throws a defiant glance at Lou.

"I can't stand the pressure any more," Lou slumps in her seat. "It's always, *when* do I want to make love? Why am I not in the mood right now? It's Sunday morning and we have no other plans, so what's wrong with me? Always why, why? I don't know. There is no reason, really. Do you think we should separate?"

There is a silence.

"It's all *your* fault then?" I ask.

Lou shrugs, resigned. Annie looks vindicated.

I wait a beat. I ask: "Doesn't it take two to tango?"

Mariushka and Sybil are in their thirties. Mariushka is an actress, Sybil works in the office of a record producer. They both like to wear leather; Sybil has a few delicate piercings in one ear, nostril, and eyebrow; Mariushka sports a butterfly tatooed below her collarbone. They met at a gay and lesbian film festival almost four years ago.

"We didn't believe in that old wives' tale, like women have sex for a year or two and then, Bye-bye, baby!" Mariushka begins. "Our encounter was so charged, we had such great sex, such passion. We were sure it would last forever."

"We would make it last," Sybil nods fiercely. "We wanted to prove it. Show everyone what bullshit that bed death thing is."

"My whole life has been a string of passionate affairs," Mariushka says. "I felt I was kind of an expert or something.

But now we're like everyone else! It's so frigging unfair."

"Perhaps we overdid it," Sybil ponders. "We did everything, you know, lingerie and toys and strap-ons... S/M and sex parties and drugs and ... what else did we do, hon?"

"Polyamorous edgeplay," Mariushka, the expert, sums it up with a toss of her long, hennaed curls.

"Yeah, and separate vacations!" Sybil adds with comic despair. "That did me in. We're exhausted, I guess. It's like it's work now. Sex has become work, you know, and it's becoming harder and harder to —"

"— get it up!" Mariushka fills in with a rueful grin. "I hate this."

"We have to take a lot of drugs these days to have good sex," Sybil wrinkles her nose with its diamond stud. "We'll end up as junkies if we keep it up. But even if we keep getting high it won't help, that's clear now. We want to know from you if there isn't anything else we could try."

"And if there isn't, I'm gonna shoot myself!" Mariushka sounds like an actress in a B movie.

Birds of a Feather

These two couples obviously represent two ends of the spectrum: "No sex and it doesn't work" on one end, and "Too much sex and it doesn't work" on the other. In between, we find the well-known sexual malaise of long-term relationships between

women. It certainly is a puzzle. In our culture, women are groomed and socially trained for relationships, but when it comes to sex — which is, after all, the most intimate form of relating — we are still stumbling across Freud's "dark continent," repeating his insistent question, "What do women want?"

We hardly know ourselves as sexual beings — which doesn't mean we aren't interested in sex. Quite the contrary. Naomi Wolf points out in her book *Promiscuities* that female sexuality was not always a dark continent. Other time periods and other cultures celebrated and had specific conceptions of the great elemental force of women's sexuality and orgasm. Two thousand years ago, Wolf reports, the Taoists of ancient China accorded female desire "the care that we now focus on the ecosystems that keep us alive and well." In our culture and time, by contrast, women and sex represent a profoundly uneasy equation; even more so, of course, if we add homosexuality to the formula.

We are aware by now that many lesbians feel the stigma and suffer the internalized homophobia of our society: The secret voice inside that whispers that same-sex desires and doings are unnatural and dirty. But if we are honest with ourselves we also know that ambivalence about sex is the cultural inheritance of all women, lesbian, bisexual, and heterosexual. Ever since Eve took her bite from the apple, women have been discouraged from acquiring sexual knowledge. We and our bodies have been seen as the dangerous seat of eros, a potentially subversive force. We have been discouraged from taking control of our bodies. We have even been discouraged from liking our bodies, thanks to the fashion and beauty dictates of our culture. And today, in our brave new twenty-first

century, there is still the powerful old moral code: Any woman with an outright appetite for sex risks being seen as a slut, while men pursue sex as their birthright — casual sex, anonymous sex, daily sex, obsessive sex, pornographic sex, etc. Women, according to the same inherited gender division, still hold the monopoly on intimacy.

Let's take a minute to trace intimacy as a female theme. We don't have to go far into gender studies and early infant development to get to some of the roots. Generally infants are taken care of by women, and thus the dominant figure for all beginning life is a woman: The all-powerful provider, the creator and destroyer in one, the Mother (with a capital M!). In a society that stresses gender differences, girls are generally raised with a heightened sense of being the same as mother; boys, by contrast, with a sense of being other. *Same as mother* means in close relation, imitating, emulating the caretaker, identifying with her.

Being birds of a feather has its shadow, however. It can mean being too close, in someone else's skin, feeling their feelings, thinking their thoughts, and finishing their sentences. It can lead to a high degree of what psychology calls merging: Loss of a separate identity and private inner space within the couple. Or, as Gloria Steinem expressed it, "I still have the female psychological disease of knowing what other people are feeling better than knowing what I'm feeling."

The "female disease" Steinem talks about is a lack of boundaries that may explain why many women seem more at ease with partners who are more "masculine" in their emotional make-up — and not just because opposites attract. Difference can be reassuring when there is an unconscious need for dis-

tance, inner space, or boundaries, although women with this kind of relationship typically complain of a lack of intimacy. On the other hand, there are lesbians who are attracted primarily by sameness. Do they have a lot more or a lot better sex in their long-term relationships? If we are honest we have to admit that none of these arrangements seem to produce or guarantee those lasting vibrations most of us are after. There must be something for us to learn.

On Dangerous Ground

Let's look a little more closely at the sexual relationship of our first couple: Annie, who feels too young to renounce sex, and Lou, whose fault it all is because she is never in the mood.

I ask Annie in the fifth session what she does when she feels turned on. How does she try to get Lou interested?

"I do everything I can," Annie says. "I prepare a special meal or bring her a mug of coffee in the morning. I look at her in a certain way, I dress a certain way... like in bed, I surprise her when she comes back from the bathroom by being without my nightgown all of a sudden...." She looks at me expectantly.

"Yes, and then?"

"I move a certain way, I move very close to her, kiss her, I even take her hand and put it on my body and sigh, or I hug her and we roll around so she gets to lie on top of me... I say things, you know... something sexy, how I love her touch...."

Or I remind her, I whisper in her ear about her favorite fantasy —about making out in a car in public...." She quickly glances at Lou to make sure she hasn't given away too much. "I mean, I try to seduce her."

"It sounds hard to resist," I propose.

"Yes," Lou suddenly comes out of her slump, "but it can also be quite annoying!"

Annie looks at her in shock over this sudden vehemence.

"It's not that I don't love her...." Lou nervously strokes her short hair. "In the beginning, this was the biggest turn-on for me. How sexy Annie was, and how I felt like I was the greatest lover on earth because of her being this way... so receptive and having so much pleasure and all."

"That was a surprise for you?" I ask.

"I've never been with anyone as femme as Annie. Most women I've known were kind of both, or tried to be. In the old movement days all of us had to be equal, remember? Counting strokes."

"And — in your experience — was it equal?"

"Of course not. I often pretended, to tell you the truth. I faked orgasm — with women! A lot! But I *gave* women a lot of orgasms, and they were not fake, I can tell you that." Lou doesn't come across as depressed and apologetic any more.

"You never told me that," Annie says, looking slightly alarmed.

"Well, no. I was afraid that I would have to do it again...."

"Fake orgasms — with me?" Annie sounds more alarmed.

"No, no! I'm only saying it's always been kind of hard for me to come. I don't like to lose control." She shifts uncomfortably on the sofa. "I'm just much more butch, I guess. At least that's what I told myself when I met Annie. I took the initiative, always, and there we were — kismet, if you like. She was

the greatest femme on earth, and I, well, I had the easy role."
She smiles apologetically again, but then bangs her fist on her
thigh. "I've been damn good at that butch role, and I know it."

"Do you agree?" I ask Annie.

"A match made in heaven," she sighs and turns to Lou. "If
it's so easy for you, why did you stop? Why don't you enjoy
it any more?"

Lou shrugs and Annie throws up her hands with impatience. I invite Annie to describe what it's like now that paradise
seems lost.

"Lou seems to resent my orgasms now," Annie explains.
"She stops before I have really come down, which normally
takes me a few orgasms. She doesn't seem with it any more.
There's this morose silence, as if I'd done something wrong.
But she won't tell me. Sometimes when I try to seduce her
now, I feel really weird, as if she judges me for being so femme
and sex-crazed or something. She doesn't like it, I feel, so I
better hold back, and then I, too, don't like it any more." She
sends Lou a reproachful look. Lou stares at the rug. "I wait
for her to be in the mood again," Annie continues, "but she
won't take the initiative, not like before. Now, whenever I try
to turn it around, I get nowhere."

"Yeah, because you don't know how," Lou says grimly.

Annie blushes. "What do you mean, I don't know how?"

"You don't know how to turn it around. Because you only
know one turn — on your back!"

Both of them look equally stunned by what has just been
said.

"And you," Annie suddenly comes back to life, red in the
face, "you only know one turn too: and that's on top of me!"

What is clear at this moment is that Lou and Annie have made a start in the direction of telling each other the truth. The tense form this takes is not surprising. When something has been kept locked up for a while and has begun to hurt, the sudden opening tends to come with a tearing, a certain violence. We all know this: When we let out pent-up steam, the hiss is going to be louder than we intend and the heat potentially more hurtful than we would like. That's precisely why we bite our tongue — for fear that our truth will come out with a mean hiss and hurt like hell. As long as we hold back, we feel in control. When we let our truth out, we are less in control. We often feel completely out of control. We don't know how our truth will sound, we don't know what it will do — it could be devastating, someone might get badly burned, it might be the end of everything.

But it could also be the beginning of everything. Telling the truth is an adventure, a loosening of control in order to do something daring. This is the first element truth has in common with good sex.

"Sex Is Magic"

Now, if telling the truth seems that dangerous, we can logically assume that we are up against something. Some authority sits in judgment over us, ready to condemn us. There is some ideal that we are supposed to embody, but don't. Some

secret expectation needs to be fulfilled by us. There is some magical bliss we are supposed to experience.

What we are up against, the powerful forces that keep us biting our tongue, are *myths*. Myths about sex.

Myths are beliefs we inherit from our culture of origin, our environment, our family upbringing — beliefs that are intended to shape our social behavior and attitudes. "All women are natural-born mothers." Or "Men have a strong natural sex drive, women don't." Myths are often simply false beliefs. Myths about sex and gender make heavy use of nature. They carry the headline "Tried and true since Adam and Eve," and they come with the instruction: "Take my word for it — don't even try to find out if it's really true." Not long ago, we had the myth of women's vaginal orgasm as the only orgasm that could count; and not long before that, according to Victorian myth, women had no sexual desire and no orgasm at all.

When we ask today which myths make it hard for lesbian couples to tell each other the truth in matters of sex, the following three regularly show up:

Myth 1.   She should just know. We are both women, we have the same body, therefore she should know what feels good and give me pleasure.

Myth 2.   There is no magic if I have to explain. It spoils everything — the romance, the surprise, the excitement — if I have to talk. Talking only interrupts. If I have to constantly provide her with a user's manual, forget about pleasure.

Myth 3.   Sex is an instinct, therefore it comes naturally. If it doesn't come naturally and easily, there's something

wrong with her ... or with me; there's something wrong with us as a couple, and we certainly won't have great sex by talking and jabbering.

These myths are so much part of our culture and upbringing that we may not even be aware that they are our bed companions. Powerful beliefs like these hook us into the romantic notion that sex is magic and that great sex is natural and easy, or else it's not great sex.

I propose to debunk these myths. In order to achieve truth and good sex, in my view, we have to admit to ourselves and each other the following facts:

1. Every woman's body is different. We cannot assume that we know a thing about our lover's body, especially given the little we tend to know about our own.

2. We have to let go of expecting our partner to be the magical lover with x ray eyes who reads all our secrets and knows our instruction manual by heart the minute she sets eyes on us. We can't go on waiting for our secrets to be guessed. Sex is communication. Sexual guessing games are like the lottery, where our chances to win are one in a million.

3. Nothing sexual in our culture is natural and easy, except for sex in Hollywood movies. Everything sexual in our culture — and therefore in our beds — is complicated and uneasy, and this malaise is not likely to change unless we stop buying into myths and instead begin to find and communicate our own individual truth.

Or, to put this in a more positive light, sex must be learned, and it can be. Good sex is like dancing well together: A lot of information has to be exchanged before two people, each with her own style of movement, can dance together with fluidity and grace.

I'd Rather Die than Tell Her

Exposing our private myths and secret beliefs can seem a scary proposition at first — a proposition we would rather avoid. We can take a guess now why our first couple never addressed the issue head-on: Annie, who is too young to give up on sex, and Lou, who is never in the mood any more. We can tell, for example, that there is a mythical belief at work: A truly happy couple would be in the mood to make love on a Sunday morning, and if this is not so, it's shameful shortcoming. For fear of failure as a couple, it was never spelled out between them that desire takes more than having a calendar at hand.

In the case of Mariushka, the actress, and Sybil, the record producer's assistant — the couple for whom sex has turned into relentless work — we detect a variation on the theme. Sybil and Mariushka believe gay male couples are enviable and there is something wrong with women. For them, it's the old gender bias: Men are sexual, women not. So if they

act like men, great sex should be a given. If they have the right toolbox and work the tools hard enough, there ought to be magical sex.

When things are not working the way our big myths have promised us they would, we can feel let down by our partners and by ourselves. We enter a state of depression, which we could call mute sexual misery. Our sex life is anything but a fairy tale. We take the malaise personally, can't even share it with our best friend (who is no doubt having great sex three times a night). The muteness of our misery makes our situation seem hopeless. We are defeated, judged, and condemned, by ourselves, without even a hearing. The lesbian bed death must be our fate. We get into fights, and the relief of reconciliation is short-lived. We project our malaise on small, insufferable traits in our lover that turn us off — things so small, we are embarrassed to even mention them.

And now we are suddenly supposed to 'fess up about them? Most couples coming to see me are shocked by the idea. When I see each parter alone for check-ins, I hear her protest: "You really mean I ought to tell her I can't stand her bad breath in the morning when she wants to make out? Talk about my phobia of breast hair? Tell her I'd like her to wear this special lace slip that belonged to my mother, that turns me on? Ask her to be more rough with me because I need to fantasize about men in order to come? Are you saying I ought to tell her I am holding back because I am afraid to fart? You mean I could tell her I'm hooked on massage as foreplay when she is already wildly jealous of my ex, the masseuse?"

Tell the truth...? The initial reaction tends to be: "I'd rather die. I'd rather make do with what we have. It's a bit boring,

okay, but better to have this than nothing." Or I hear: "Oh, I tried to tell her, but she doesn't get it. It's useless." Or: "I once told her, and she never forgave me. It really spoiled it all."

Okay, if this is all there is, forget it. The bad breath and snore have successfully strangled our sex life. Truth-telling would be the final blow in our bed.

This is what almost happened to Annie and Lou when their bomb went off all of a sudden in that fifth session. If they had had a choice about it, they wouldn't have blurted out their anger over their lover's role limitation in bed. Annie and Lou each felt hurt by the unexpected criticism. It took some work to undo the sense of betrayal both felt because they had been kept in the dark. This is a loaded aspect of couples' communication: When the truth is suddenly out, we can resent the betrayal of not having been told sooner.

For Annie and Lou, the perceived betrayal put them through a phase of doubt in their entire relationship. What was true and what wasn't? Had Lou really never faked her orgasms with Annie? Had Annie just pretended that everything was perfect and nothing was missing in their love life? Had they kept other secrets and criticisms from each other?

Instead of withdrawing in pain or running from the challenge, Lou and Annie managed to overcome this blow to their self-esteem through conscious effort. They found an interest in exploring who they were and how they had gotten there. This soul-searching in our sessions allowed them to take each other's sexual histories anew, from a fresh perspective. Most couples do this kind of "intake" at the beginning of their dating or commitment, of course. Doing it again, a few years later, can bring back some of the excitement of the honeymoon phase,

when telling secrets is part of the erotic energy.

Lou and Annie's moment of truth shows that the degree of shock and dismay over a sudden revelation depends on two elements: The length of time that truth has been in hiding, and the form it takes when it bursts forth without warning. How do we deal with this unpredictability? How could we prevent truth-telling from indeed being the final blow to our relationship?

As a first step, I suggest we reframe it.

A Possibility

Let's consider truth as simply a possibility, like good sex: Something worth exploring and working towards. A goal, no more, no less. The very idea of working towards, working something out, is encouraging. It softens the frightening absoluteness of the Truth with a capital T. Adrienne Rich reminds us that there is no absolute truth: Truth is "an increasing complexity."

It may also be an increasing simplicity. There are many little steps towards many little truths, leading to more and more discoveries —some complex, some simple— about who we are. A Taoist saying goes, "A journey of a thousand miles begins with one step." One step and we are on our way. Let's remember: Truth is an approach, a move towards something we wish for, something we want to change. Truth almost always brings out something we desire (there's that link again with sex).

But why is it that truth-telling so often sounds like criticism? "I really can't stand it when you…"; "I honestly wish you wouldn't always…." We recognize the ring of it, the slightly wrong note in the music: An exasperation, impatience, even something of an accusation and undercover attack. When we notice this kind of tone and wording, we might wonder: What are we covering up? Is it too risky to voice our longing, and the pain of our longing, openly?

When we criticize, we feel more safe, more defended. We talk about the other, using "you language": Language in which *you* are primarily responsible for the problem. But when we express a desire, especially a hidden desire or a painful longing, we feel vulnerable. We have to talk about ourselves and reveal something sensitive. We feel that much more is at stake. What may be at stake is, for example, a dangerous cultural taboo: Women shouldn't want anything too much. It's not the feminine thing. Having desires indicates that we are egoistical, narcissistic, needy — or, as we have already seen, a slut. We may be criticized or humiliated for our pain and longing. We may be rejected.

Whatever the underlying reasons, we can try to become aware of the difference in the "music" — the difference between the voice of our desire and the voice of our criticism. It will make a difference in our relationship. If we are on the thousand-mile journey towards truthfulness and sexual bliss, why hide from the fact that behind all our criticizing there is always wishfulness and wistfulness? Behind our attacks is a vulnerable desire for something that might bring us closer together.

So we reframe truth as something that needs to be worked on. It needs keen listening. And it needs attention to the choice

of words, the tone of voice, the "music." For what we want will have to be said out loud. Wishful thinking alone won't get us what we want. Waiting and hoping that she might guess is that lottery again, where most likely, we won't hit the jackpot. Waiting and hoping are things many women are very good at, to our own detriment. Wishful thinking, by itself, keeps us in a childlike position, caught up in magic, which means expecting to be known and understood without having to do much or even anything about it.

Let's admit it: This magical child's expectation of passive fulfillment is almost everyone's (conscious or unconscious) dream: Surprise me, do to me exactly what I long for ... give me bliss without any effort on my part. Give me the ideal mother who dispenses her heavenly milk just when the baby begins to feel the need and craving for it. Most of us seem to have a vague memory of this passive state of bliss — and if not a memory, a nostalgic longing for something that takes care of our wishes in this way. This, above all, is the magical hope we bring to sexual encounters. Here, finally, is the one, the dream lover who will know and satisfy all of my longings and desires by pure magic.

Magical encounters and nights of bliss do happen, but alas, they don't repeat in a reliable fashion, time after time and year after year. This is where Annie got caught. Lou had been her dream lover, and now Annie was waiting and hoping every Sunday that Lou would magically be in the mood again. Yes, she made some attempts to seduce Lou back into that mood, but it wasn't working. Annie became increasingly reproachful and critical of Lou. She was always in the right mood, wasn't she, and she did what she could, didn't she? Annie didn't

realize that with her silent waiting and hoping she had, in effect, relinquished her power to Lou. Like a child, she had let herself become dependent on Lou as an all-powerful provider of happiness. Annie didn't provide her own happiness, and she wasn't aware that passive dependence, no matter how blissful at moments, ends up generating resentment. Something else is needed for fulfillment.

In recent infant development studies, it has been shown that a satisfying relation between mother and infant relies on subtle cues of communication exchanged and picked up by both participants. There is no passive happy baby. That happy baby is mighty active, science has found.

Clues from Childhood

If even the infant is active and communicating, the sexual woman had better pick up a few clues. But here we find a paradox: There's nothing like having to tell our secrets and speak the truth, without criticizing, to reduce us to the state of a stuttering child. We struggle, we are scared, we are ashamed, we are awkward, tongue-tied. We draw a blank.

At this point, let's remember that we don't have to be perfect. We don't have to be good at this. We are only working towards, only learning. We are just beginners. Remember the rewards: We might get closer to what we wish for. And so we speak. We propose to our lover that she hear our secret longing

and our hidden pain. And while we tremble because we have possibly just stepped on a bomb or created an earthquake, it is surprising how often we hear: "Honey, I had no idea you felt like this, why didn't you tell me a long time ago?"

No explosion; the earth still stands. Our relationship hasn't disappeared into an abyss. Instead, a space has opened for us. We are invited into a sunlit clearing in the middle of a dark and dangerous forest, invited to say more, to reveal more of our truth: "Why didn't you tell me a long time ago?"

When Lou and Annie came to this clearing, both of them asked the same question: Why? And both at first came up with the same answer: "But I tried! I tried so many times to tell you. You just wouldn't listen."

At this point in our quest for truth, do we buy it? Our partner looks nonplussed. Tried? So many times? And she is still clueless? She usually isn't deaf. She usually loves us and has good intentions towards us. Something here doesn't gel. If we go back to the active baby, we detect a telling difference. When the baby's needs are not met, there is no doubt about it. The baby hollers and screams up a storm. The grown woman, by contrast, whispers and hints. She sends longing glances. She sulks. She exerts magical, wishful thinking and waits.

But now that she is encouraged by her lover to come forward, perhaps she will admit that she didn't dare speak up and make any serious noise about her hidden reality; that she was too shy, or too scared. The admission of being scared in the middle of a dangerous forest tends to elicit protectiveness from her lover. More room is opening up in the clearing. If she is brave enough, she will take another step forward and reveal her fear — then take a breath and find a few words that bring

her secret longing into the open at last. Then her lover may say, "I would love to, you know, but I can only do this for you if you promise not to always get half-drunk before we make love." Or she might say, "Honestly, I can't, I can't do it always, but I could try to do it more often...." And she might add, "I'll try it if you do that one special thing for me in return that I have always been ashamed to ask for...."

Truth-telling engenders creative negotiations: Creative, because it can be surprising what we are suddenly willing to give if certain conditions are met. This is the way children naturally negotiate on the playground: "I want to drive your red truck around." "Okay, if I can play with your Barbie doll." For an adult couple trying to negotiate difficult needs and wants, it can be a great relief to approach it like kids on a playground.

Most women have been taught early on to be giving, to be selfless, to always put the other's needs first. There is no doubt in my mind that the giving of gifts is one of the essential expressions of lovingness. Some women see giving as profoundly linked to women's nature and our capacity to give birth. True as this may be, *wanting* to give and *having* to give are worlds apart. Women's assigned "duties" of selflessness tend to create painful confusions and resentments, especially in feminist and so-called postfeminist times, when women are also supposed to be affirmative about their own needs. Going back to the sandbox, where we can openly declare and question who gives what to whom and how much, can clear out a lot of these confusions and silent resentments.

And it doesn't necessarily devalue our gift to be rewarded with something we desire for ourselves. If you watch little kids at play, you may notice that handing over that precious red

truck can still very much be felt as gift-giving, even if the Barbie doll is received in return.

Naming and negotiating rewards for what we are willing to give or give up make it that much easier to show each other little bits of our naked self. "I'm so embarrassed, you know I'm uptight about oral sex, but if you got me real excited, you know, if you'd whisper in my ear and, you know, use your tongue and all, I think I could get in the mood for it and really like doing it...." When we see and experience how scared, ashamed, and vulnerable we both are, often empathy comes, and so does tenderness. We are moved, and a certain innocence is restored. We are again, for a moment, like children who can simply say, I hurt, I want, I need.

That's a very different child from the one who broods and secretly waits for magical guesses. This is the creative child who dares to engage the other — the lover — through self-expression, through open and direct wanting, through truth. When our hearts open in this way, the walls between us melt away. So does the body armor that has held our fear and resentment and kept us at arm's length. The body resonates with the tenderness of the heart and opens; it wants to hug, touch, lie down and offer itself.

Truth-making and lovemaking have a lot in common. Think of the powerful impulse when we are newly in love, attracted to someone: We are overcome by desire, a desire so strong that it can triumph over all obstacles and inhibitions in order to express itself. The pressure of longing that builds up inside guides us to take it outside, where it comes out, where we come out. The same is true with truth: A similar buildup of tension, desire, fear, and wanting develops that in the end guides us to

find expression. And when it's found, that right word — the relief can be like an orgasm! We all know how great it can feel, this refreshing, delicious moment of truth.

The Coolest Game

A moment like this came up in an early session with Mariushka and Sybil, the couple who had tried every device to safeguard their sexual magic. Mariushka and Sybil are describing their relationship to me. They are particularly proud of the fact that from the start, they gave each other permission to look at and flirt with other women.

"If you are only two and you are only looking at each other, how boring after a time," Mariushka proclaims. "I mean, where's the inspiration supposed to come from, the juice? Beauty is such a turn-on. And if you don't flirt, you dry out, you forget that you are a sexual being."

She is getting more fiery by the second. I notice that while Sybil listens and nods at Mariushka's diatribe, her eyes look dead. I ask her what she is feeling at this moment.

"This is so important to Mariushka," she says. "I am sometimes not in the mood to flirt with some stranger, but I know Mariushka finds it a big turn-on when I do. She's the actress. So I go along with it."

"You mean you flirt with other women because Mariushka wants you to?"

"Oh, it's fun, of course, once I get into it," she says.

"What would happen if you didn't get into it, if you followed only your own mood?"

"I'm always in the mood," she says, then laughs, as if her words sound too unlikely to her own ears. "That's what I am supposed to be." She glances at Mariushka. "What would happen? I'll tell you the truth: Then Mariushka would be the only one flirting around and I would hate that. I would feel so excluded. I already often feel I am just not enough for her, and then I feel hurt and jealous when she is staring at other women...."

"So you flirt, too, in order not to feel those feelings?"

She nods, looking nervous.

"But honey," Mariushka jumps out of her chair, kneels down at Sybil's side and takes her hand with a flourish. "I thought this was fun for you! You always seem to be so turned on by other women. You give me the impression that this is the coolest game we have. I play the game for you!"

"For me?!" Sybil looks at her in disbelief.

"Believe me!" Mariushka says. "I don't need this! Tell me to stop, I'll stop."

"But I thought you only love me when I do this far-out stuff," Sybil says. "That you only desire me when I am openly sexual...in public. If I didn't you wouldn't find me interesting, I feel. You wouldn't pay attention to me."

"Funny thing is," Mariushka is suddenly thoughtful, "I'm not always in the mood either, you know? But you often look somehow...bored or absent or something, and then I feel I have to make an effort to cheer you up and turn you on and get a game going."

"You make an effort? To turn me on?" Sybil seems stunned.

Mariushka shrugs. "It's true. I really do it for you more than for myself. I do it for us. I'm afraid you'd be bored if I didn't constantly…"

There is a silence.

"So both of you do a lot of things for each other — not because you truly desire them, but because you think the other wants them or needs them?" I ask.

"But that's absurd!" Sybil looks at Mariushka, who is still kneeling beside her, and starts laughing. "Are you sure?"

They both laugh uproariously until it suddenly becomes clear that Sybil's laughter has turned into tears.

"I'm so tired of it," she sobs. "So fucking tired… of fucking."

And then they both roar again with laughter.

In this breakthrough moment for Sybil and Mariushka, the truth came as a surprise and brought instant relief to them both. Less surprisingly, this one incident of truth-finding became the trigger that encouraged the couple to look further and find similar patterns of trying to please each other that were burdening their relationship.

Wanting to do our lover a favor, wanting to please, not wanting to disappoint: These are loving, caring impulses that can all too easily trap women if truth-telling does not sufficiently come into the equation. We may get stuck in one of the big myths or merely a big assumption: She wants this, she needs it, she will be bored with me if I don't, she will think I don't love her if I refuse, etc. And the assumption is never spelled out, let alone questioned. We are too scared to call for a reality check, because that would reveal some of our true feelings and concerns. "We dance round in a ring and suppose," said the poet

Robert Frost, "but the Secret sits in the middle and knows...."

When Mariushka and Sybil began to unravel the truth of what they were doing for each other without really wanting to do it, it became clear why they were so tired of their relationship and why sex had become work.

Likewise, when Annie, who felt too young to renounce sex, and Lou, whose fault it all was, discovered their resentments about their rigid role division, it became clear why there was no sexual appetite any more between them.

And now what? Most couples complain at this stage that telling the truth and gaining an understanding of a problem does not automatically solve it. They sometimes get frustrated and angry with the process, accusing me of making it all worse for them. Understanding a problem can make one very nervous, and that's a good reason many people stay away from it. Understanding brings the sudden realization that we have to do something about the situation. We have to change.

If Lou and Annie want to do something about it, they have to face changing sexual roles, which they have carefully avoided doing because they don't know how. If Mariushka and Sybil want to change, they have to limit what they do with each other to what they really desire, and they don't know if there is anything they still desire.

Both couples tell me they feel lost and scared. How are they going to do this?

Now What?

Think about it for a moment. Have you had many good teachers who showed you how to tell the truth? Frankly, I haven't. There certainly were lots of voices about the virtue of truth, there were parental admonitions, puritanical warnings, some wise pronouncements from philosophers and spiritual teachers. But no *how-to*. No "Easy Steps to Telling the Truth," although everybody seems to agree that it isn't easy. It's especially hard for women, who hate to hurt anybody's feelings. So how do we study it and learn it? Nobody tells us.

Here we have another parallel with sex — although you might argue that in matters of sex, we have plenty of information. Ever since Plato's *Symposium,* there has been a literature describing, and thus teaching, sex. There have been erotica and pornography for ages, there have been Chaucer, Casanova, and the Marquis de Sade. Ever since the Victorian Age ended, there hasn't been a single corner of the bed that hasn't been turned over and examined for another how-to sex manual. In the last few decades, we have progressed from *The Joy of Sex* to Pat Califia's *Sapphistry* and *Bitch Goddess* to Carol Queen's *The Leather Daddy and the Femme.* Is there anything we don't know?

We have learned from the Kinsey Report, Masters and Johnson, and *The Hite Report;* we don't fear any more that masturbation will cause brain damage; we have had R-rated and X-rated movies, porn magazines at the corner store; we've been getting *Behind the Green Door* and down the *Deep Throat;* we've read *Lolita* and *The Story of O;* we've followed the latest fads: The G-spot, ecstasy, tantric workshops — but what if all this hasn't taught us much or anything about our individual sexual

selves, our own mysterious sexual bodies? Could it be that sex and truth can't be taught? Wouldn't it be amazing if after a hundred years of sexual experimentation, sexual liberation, and sexual revolution; after birth control and the Summer of Love; after taking back our bodies and the night — we still don't know much more about sex than the Victorians did?

It is a provocative thought. I would argue that throughout these sexual liberations, we have also been taught to ignore and violate our bodies. We have taught our bodies to silence our voices about our inclinations and fears, while we have strived to be or act like the liberated woman of our time: Thinner, freer, sexier by the decade. Many of us have forced our bodies into risky experiments and whipped them into sexual frenzies. We have set out to conquer the "dark continent." We have taken our lovers and ourselves to the edge and back. Yet we are still puzzled and lost. We are still asking the same questions about how to reach a lover and be reached, how to communicate love through sex and sustain passion in a love relationship. In her book *Ferocious Romance*, the well-known leather dominatrix Donna Minkowitz expresses precisely this profound state of puzzlement and dissatisfaction: "I've found one of the loves of my life, and the only way that I can touch her is with variously stinging bits of leather." There is the sadness of wondering: How come it's so often been in vain when we have tried so hard?

Well, what if our cries and whispers of wanting are an alphabet that we ourselves have to continue to learn — the secret alphabet of our bodies that we have to help each lover master? We grow, our bodies change, we age. With every new life phase this alphabet may have to be spelled out again. With every new relationship, a new language of the body may have to be

found and spoken, patiently and passionately, if we want to be sexually uncovered, found, and finally fulfilled.

It is hard to fulfill a desire we ourselves do not know.

But let's not give up. Let's remember we are on a journey. Let's contemplate this Japanese haiku, with its sexy subtext:

> *Yes, snail,*
> *climb Mount Fuji,*
> *but slowly, slowly.*

There is no denying that the snail at the foot of the mountain may be tempted to give up.

"What is it with this whole sex thing?" Lou asked in one of our earlier sessions. "Who says it's all that important anyway?" Before Annie has a chance to reply that it's important to *her*, Lou launches into a diatribe.

"Sex is just another industry," she maintains, "a consumer product like any other. Do we need fifteen different toilet papers? Most of what we are supposed to need, we don't need at all. And now we need to have sex. Fifteen times a week! And along with it, fifteen magazines about seduction and climaxing, and what not, and books, and sex films, and lingerie… all that nonsense. Does anyone ask us if we even want this?" She flashes glances around the room. "I don't!" she declares defiantly just as Annie quietly says, "I do.…"

Annie read Wilhelm Reich in the seventies, and his theories of orgasm convinced her that sex is healthy and the quality of orgasm matters.

"It's good for you," she decrees. "The entire organism needs orgasm to get back into balance. Energy flow, the juices, you know? If nature gives it, why not take it?"

"Yeah, like we are trees with their sap. If we have urges, fine. We can do it ourselves. Nature has given us just the right length of arms, no? Isn't that funny? But from there to go into that sex craze, and put it on a throne, like Reich did? No way. I'll soon be in menopause anyway, and what matters to me is that we can be close without it. We love each other. We are very happy with our lives. Why add pressure?"

"Why add pleasure?" Annie quips.

This gets us into an interesting discussion on what sex is. And what is it good for? I notice that Annie seems to have fun driving a strong argument and cornering Lou whenever she can; and that Lou repeats herself and gets befuddled, but she eyes Annie with secret glee. I can tell that she is not really intent on winning the game. She enjoys the fact that Annie is playing a power game and giving the ball a good kick.

The talk turns more emotional when Annie declares, "Okay, sex is not a must-have, but it makes a difference. A big one for me. I love you, true, and I feel we are close. But when we make love, something else happens. How to describe it? I adore you. I suddenly feel all the walls give way, all the struggles and quibbles between us are gone, poof! Blown away, forgotten. Only love is there, and some enormous gratitude. I could do anything for you at that moment. I feel I belong to you, with every fiber. I give you everything I have and everything I am. It's yours."

After their fighting and debating, this is a moment of great intensity. Lou is smitten, I can tell. She is swayed. She can't help but agree that Annie is right. Sex, for Lou, is still worth a try.

Back to Square One

To be sure, the slow climb up Mount Fuji is a journey into the unknown. But it is good to remember that this scary feeling of the unknown is based on something only partly real. Annie and Lou, Mariushka and Sybil already know a lot of things: They have begun to tell the truth; they have entered a negotiation to get what they want; and of course, they do know something about what they do or do not desire. So there's in fact a lot of knowledge to start with. And now we discover that *not* knowing something may be the most reassuring fact of all.

It is an enormous relief for a couple to be able to say, "We both want this, we want to have love and sexual satisfaction in our relationship, but we don't know how to go about it." It's a revelation. It's two lovers admitting to each other the simple truth that all of us are the products of a culture that forces us to know everything about sex while it teaches us nothing. All of a sudden there is a chance to be young again, and to declare openly and without shame: "I have to learn everything. I don't know how to seduce you, how to take you, I don't know how to give up control to you, I don't know how to say no when you touch me, I don't know how to tell you how to do it right...." We are making our way back to our innocence, where little is known and nothing can be assumed. We are committing to a fresh slate where, as a couple, we have permission and relative safety to experiment and find out. That

shared mental space where nothing is assumed and truth can be told, is what I call "Love's Learning Place."

We all know this place. When we fall in love and begin to make love we are perhaps not aware that we are at a "learning place," discovering what we like and dislike as lovers, what sexually pleases or frightens us. As a newly forming couple, we engage in this process naturally. But when our implicit agreement, our couple arrangement doesn't work sexually or doesn't work any more, another phase begins. Usually this is a volatile phase. There are fights and frustrations, and the temptation to throw in the towel. Often couples seek therapy at this stage.

Instead of seeing such an impasse as a failure, I see it as an unavoidable passage in any long-term relationship. The challenge of this passage is change, breaking out of old habits, refining truth, and redefining the couple. When lovers engage in some couples work at this point, they are consciously reentering Love's Learning Place. Instead of being embarrassed at having fallen from paradise, they may find that they are on a lovers' journey back. When our big myths have failed us, instead of being ashamed of our sexual shortcomings, we can find erotic liberation by reentering Love's Learning Place.

This strategy worked for Annie and Lou. It encouraged them to paint a clear and honest picture of their couple dynamic in bed. It became clear that Lou felt frustrated by Annie's hogging the receiving role, always playing the femme. But Lou couldn't play that feminine role because she was too scared to give over control. Therefore she never really asked Annie to take the active role, but secretly resented her lover

for her lack of "butch" skills. By resisting Annie's seductions, she tried to provoke Annie to change and come on to her, which Annie didn't dare do. Now the full picture revealed that both lovers were afraid to shift roles, and afraid to address the fact squarely.

When a couple decides to share the blame, blame tends to fall away altogether. Without blaming, we can consider experimenting and searching for solutions...together.

This is what Annie and Lou did. Hand in hand, so to speak, they reentered what they now called Love School, and thought out a plan to get out of their sexual impasse. They playfully decided they were already in second grade at Love School, because they had successfully mastered one role constellation. This achievement was not to be abandoned, because now that the truth was out and there was hope for something new, Lou felt less resentful about that old role division. It would still be fun to play butch–femme the easy way. Second grade, however, was about learning to add the opposite roles to their repertoire. Lou now had to play "femme," which meant she had to tolerate Annie's shy and clumsy attempts at playing Don Juan. This wasn't easy for the two, and often hysterical laughing attacks from either one made any concentration or romantic, sexy mood impossible. Even being serious did not bring them great results at first, and again, they had to face the challenge of telling each other the truth about it.

In our sessions, I pointed out to them that their talks about control and power were deepening. Lou and Annie were now looking closely at other power divisions in their life. The story they had lived by and told me when they first came in, that they were equally in love with their computer business and

had the same golf handicap, began to sound a little different. It turned out that Lou, who was tired of having to be butch in bed, played a patronizing, "fatherly" role in their business, secretly keeping Annie out of important decisions. On the golf course, she let Annie win half the time because she felt protective of Annie's vulnerability. Open competition was uncomfortable for Lou, so she hid her advantage and secretly kept Annie in the one-down, "femme" position.

But was Annie really in need of Lou's protection? It turned out that as a child, Annie had adopted a certain "feminine" fragility as a way to placate an aggressively critical father. Being seductive and unchallenging had been her way of protecting herself. As a feminist, however, and in her relationship with Lou, Annie had been trying to clean up her act and bravely pretend that "we are all strong and equal now." But she let Lou protect her, and sexually, she didn't dare take on an active role.

Once Annie and Lou understood how they had both played into this pattern, changes could be worked out. Lou agreed to give Annie more room to assert herself, both in their business and in their private life. She supported Annie's overcoming her handicaps. In their business and on the golf course, Annie struggled to discover her healthy ambitions, while Lou tried to cope with her fear that in any open competition she would overwhelm her lover and end up alone. Both partners frequently felt unnerved by their own courage, but they also felt pride and a growing compassion for each other as a result of these talks and new challenges.

The Helpmate

Progress in bed was slower, and there was a period when impatience almost got the better of them. Lou discovered the essay "The Uses of Anger," by the late poet Audre Lorde, and put a quote from it on the fridge. It read, "We cannot allow our fear of anger to deflect us nor seduce us into settling for anything less than the hard work of excavating honesty." Annie countered with a handwritten note saying, "Less work, more play!" The couple experienced the well-known fact that after a good fight, sex can suddenly be good, too.

What do sex and fights have to do with each other? Lou and Annie found that their fights allowed them to come out with some more truth. Not necessarily *the Truth* with a capital T, they discovered, because anger tends to blow everything out of proportion. But airing bottled-up resentment in these angry confrontations created a release and brought the relief of distance between them. Annie and Lou found that out of this experience of more distance and independence, a new desire and energy for closeness could arise.

Annie got more feisty and gradually was more in the mood to try to "take" her lover. But Lou wouldn't let her. Lou had a hard time being on the receiving end, and she was not very motivated to understand her own conditioning. "That's just my nature," Lou would argue. Now it was Annie's turn to put a quote from Audre Lorde on the fridge: "What understanding begins to do is to make knowledge available for use,

and that's the urgency, that's the push, that's the drive." And indeed, Annie developed urgency, push, and drive to understand Lou's resistance.

Little by little, Lou's fear of receiving pleasure began to make sense through childhood memories. Lou had learned early on to renounce her own needs and pleasures in order to protect and please a demanding, vulnerable mother who would punish her with silent withdrawal. From childhood on, Lou had had to be very much in control of herself in order to avert abandonment by her mother. When Lou got in touch with this knowledge, with her childhood self, she cried a lot, and Annie loved to hold her. Annie began to feel protective of Lou, and one day, her compassion for Lou's difficulties inspired her.

"You need a helpmate, sweetheart," she suddenly announces in session.

Lou looks puzzled.

"Remember Adam?" Annie helps her along. "He, too, couldn't do it alone. So God gave him a helpmate, right?" She fumbles in her bag and retrieves a package wrapped in a brown paper bag.

Lou starts when she unwraps her gift — an elegant little vibrator.

"It's a Ladyfinger," Annie says encouragingly. "A toy."

"Yeah, but I'm not a baby... I don't like toys," Lou says and hides the thing back in its bag.

Annie's face falls.

"Have you tried any adult toys?" I ask Lou.

She shakes her head. "It's yucky somehow. I don't want to try."

"You haven't tried any," I ponder. "That must be hard, I imagine,

once again to be asked to try out something new that you have no experience with. To take on the role of the fool, so to speak, for everyone to see. For Annie to see...."

"But I don't know any better than you do," Annie rushes in to assure Lou. "Do you think I have ever used one? I'm a fool too! That's why I got this." She fishes a videotape out of her bag and holds it up for us. "See? All you ever wanted to know about toys but never dared to ask. Scary. So we can put the lights out, hold hands and shudder together while we watch it. Huuuhhhu!"

Lou can't help grinning, but she is not convinced. The three of us talk at length about Lou's notion that taking a vibrator to bed is an admission of failure. Many lesbians consider using a tool like a vibrator a particularly shameful failure, because it means that women can't have sex without a penis-presence in bed. Even though Lou sees through this and laughs her head off at the notion that women need anything men have, she still isn't comfortable with this "penis-presence." Annie, who has turned feisty, exchanges her Ladyfinger for a regular massage wand that shows no risky resemblance to any body part.

Now the next myth comes out of the closet: Only honest, hard work deserves to be rewarded by pleasure. There is no honest, hard work with a joystick.

We talk some more about the puritanical creed that we can have pleasure solely as a reward for laboring or fulfilling some duty; that pleasure is not supposed to be a gift in itself, even a God-given gift. We talk about the notion of play — for example, in playing golf. Lou understands the difference between a stiff, belabored swing and a relaxed, playful swing. She knows the latter has a better chance to be pleasurable and successful,

to boot. We discuss playfulness as a highly desirable part of all human activity, especially sports and sex. The golf analogy does the trick: Lou agrees to try out "that thing" — but only in private and only for her shoulder aches! Soon afterwards, however, the thing is assigned a role in Lou and Annie's lovemaking: It is now the "putter" that gets Lou's ball across the last few inches into the hole when Lou has the handicap of playing "femme".

So Annie's idea worked in the end. Knowing that Lou could use the toy any time she needed to be in control of her own pleasure was the right strategy. It allowed both of them to be less anxious about their tasks in Love's Learning Place.

"We have a new name for it," Annie reports a few sessions later. "We call it Play Practice now."

Lou nods. "I always used to be so nervous about would I come, and how long would it take me to come. I mean, that's why I used to fake orgasms. I was embarrassed. The longer it took the more I was sure I would never come, and with Annie I'd rather renounce my orgasm and pretend it wasn't that important for me. But with that little putter," she grins at Annie, "I don't have to worry any more. I score. And Annie doesn't have to work too hard either. All because of Good Vibrations, the Little Store That Could!"

"How do you feel about this?" I ask Annie.

"I'm not so sure that I am not a little bit jealous here," Annie says with a mock growl. "I'm doing the work and I don't see the effect because our helpmate comes onto the scene and steals the show!"

"Oh, don't give me that!" Lou pouts. "It's your fault. You gave that thing to me. You made me." They both look at me

from the corners of their eyes to check if I will buy this.

"Poor Lou," I say. "Poor Annie."

Shortly after this session, Lou and Annie began to do what they called "weaning" themselves from counseling. They felt they knew enough to be on their own. After their termination, we kept a schedule of check-ins at first, then I heard only sporadically that things were going well for the two of them and that Lou hardly ever declined an invitation for sex on a Sunday morning.

Now, did this mean they had graduated to the capacity for changing roles? Interestingly, no. But through their patient trying out and finding solutions, Annie and Lou discovered an entirely new dimension to their lovemaking that they had not expected: A caring that led to an intimate sense of being together and feeling more equal in bed. The clever use they made of their helpmate allowed them not to care so much about who was active and who was passive, but instead, to hold each other, hugging and kissing and fondling — while coming, with relative ease, together. In the last message I received, I learned that Annie and Lou were weathering the turbulence of menopause quite well, thanks to their continued Play Practice.

Polymorphously Perverse

In my work with many couples over the years, I have found that people find their own name for their own version of Love's

Learning Place. LLP, Play Practice, Love School, Love Journey, Love Temple, and Initiation Place are a few of them. When a couple manages to make the concept their own, a lot has been gained. A good sexual relationship — just like a good relationship on the whole — is life-long learning. Nobody passes a final exam in life, and the same holds true in Love's Learning Place. There are no grades, although a couple mastering a problem of sexual frustration may feel like they have just graduated, even summa cum laude. There are no teachers other than one's lover, although there may be the counselor or guide on the outside who helps the couple maintain the spirit. That spirit is the honest realization that we know little or next to nothing about sex to begin with. For even if we proclaim ourselves great lovers, it takes two to tango. If you have watched people on a dance floor, you may have noticed how easily a novice can cause a first-class dancer to lose her step, or how a rumba master and a champion of Viennese waltzes may make an awkward, inhibited pair. If these two want to find pleasure dancing with each other they will have to begin again, together.

That's more or less what Mariushka and Sybil set out to do — the two "pros" who had lost the taste for sex. They couldn't get it up any more, as Mariushka had joked. Their problem was that sex was not really a communication between them; it was a performance for the other, with each lover assuming that's what the other wanted, admired, and applauded.

After a short number of sessions, Sybil and Mariushka were ready to admit that there was something artificial in their sex life, but the distinction between real passion and make-believe seemed lost. It was much harder for this couple to face the truth and do something about it because there seemed to

be a little bit of make-believe in everything they were used to doing. And as they were already working too hard on their sexual relationship, the very idea of going back to a place of learning rubbed them the wrong way.

"That's like school, like kindergarten," Mariushka protests. "I've always hated school, and I've cheated and flunked most of the time. The whole idea is a turn-off, to tell you the truth."

"I'm glad you are telling me the truth," I say. "You are welcome to laugh about it. Call it Sandbox. The funnier the name the better. Experimenting and trying something new should be fun, not a punishment."

"Could we call it Sex Camp?" Sybil tries to be cheerful. "Although I don't know what new tricks we'd have left to learn in there, after what we've been through...."

"I am not a sex therapist," I remind her, "nor is this sex therapy. It's precisely the learning place for *love*, because there you are — sexperts so to speak, with diplomas and a big toolbox — but you are not generating happiness with all that. You are tired and exasperated, you told me, instead of feeling more love for each other. So, if the old tricks aren't working any more, why not try a new approach?"

They look at me skeptically.

"How long has it been since you two have held hands, looked into each other's eyes for a while, and felt moved by tenderness?"

"Oh no," Mariushka moans, "I see you coming. Instead of sex, you want us to do tickle-tickle under the covers, in the dark. Snore! Lesbian bed death guaranteed! That's exactly what we wanted to avoid, don't you see?"

When Mariushka and Sybil opened up and described their

ways of making out, I noticed a frantic, formalized quality to their sex. Lovemaking for them resembled staged theater acts. There was make-up, costumes, setting the stage. There was very little spontaneous playfulness, hardly ever laughter. Apart from ritualized turn-on language and buzzwords, they did not talk to each other during sex. When I commented on the limitation and emotional paucity of these exchanges, Sybil and Mariushka were dumbstruck. They had been so proud of their achievements. Now Mariushka protested that I wanted to turn them into "lame vanilla lesbians."

Over the next sessions, we had a lively discussion about what sex is and what isn't. Is a foot massage sex? Is a backrub sex? Is hugging sex? To Mariushka, all this was "vanilla nonsense"; to her, sex and tenderness were incompatible. But Sybil gradually expressed a growing interest in something she now felt she had probably missed.

"It's like we have this image in our heads to be like men," she ponders one day, "like, men know how to do it. Their sex is better. And it's best when it's anonymous sex. Sex with a stranger."

"But it's true," Mariushka interrupts. "With a stranger, you feel the real adventure, the risk...."

"Maybe," Sybil concedes. "But we are not strangers. Only, we pretend we are. I mean, we make this effort all the time to be something else, something we want to be, instead of who we really are."

"But who are we?" Mariushka wants to know.

Sybil is silent.

"Are you saying that parts of yourself, certain feelings or needs can't be expressed? There's no room for them?" I ask.

"Yes, like, I can't be weak or needy or childlike — that's not okay, that's taboo. We always have to be so tough and independent and bitchy, and that creates this odd distance, something cold, between us. How could it hurt to be a little tender every once in a while?" Sybil swallows. "I sometimes wish...I could be clingy...and be held, and feel safe."

Mariushka looks at her with big, surprised eyes. She seems about to object, glances at me, looks back at Sybil. There is no argument. Sybil has revealed a secret. She has touched a sensitive spot.

From there, we went on to explore what it means to follow an image, to worship an ideal instead of appreciating what's real. Whether it's movie sex idols or men, the idealized image carries the magical expectation that hooks us and keeps us from experiencing and communicating our true wishes and needs. The prefabricated sexual image of how we ought to be, and now want to be, keeps us from discovering who we are. Adopting a "male" sexuality may be an exciting game for a while. But we can't grow, learn, or develop within a stereotype. We remain frozen in a repetition that soon loses all life.

It took Sybil and Mariushka a while to unravel their sexual beliefs and question their myths. In the end, Sybil's need for tenderness prevailed, and Mariushka gave in ... with a sigh.

"Okay, back to the sandbox. What do we have to lose?"

They demanded some homework. Their task was to notice what they were doing when they had sex, and to notice what they were feeling while doing it. I called their attention to frustrations, emptiness, childlike longings, the sense of forcing themselves or feeling forced. Very quickly, even Mariushka was struck by the lack of gentleness in their relationship.

Caressing, they began to realize, always had an ulterior motive. It wasn't enough in itself as a way of giving and receiving simple pleasure. It had to lead up to the big bang of the orchestrated climax, and then to another one, as fast as possible.

"How about not having sex for a while?" I suggest one day when the couple is caught in angry blaming of each other for not doing things right and feeling bored.

Both of them stare at me in shock.

"You want us to work on a sexual problem by giving up sex?" Mariushka asks. "Next, we'll do homework with a chastity belt!"

"Well, there's an idea," I say. "But abstinence in itself is not good enough. As you well know from your separate vacations, after a break one tends to be very quickly back to square one. Unless something essential has changed ... in the sandbox."

"Oh no," they moan in chorus, "what do we have to do now?"

Together, we make a list of all the things that can be done in a sandbox, like touching, looking, examining, tasting, counting strokes, etc. — but no sex. That will be the rule. I call it being polymorphously perverse, and that notion hits home.

Polymorphous perversity is a concept that Freud introduced almost a hundred years ago in order to describe children's early sexuality — a phase that he thought should and would be outgrown by the awakening of mature genital sexual desire. But we can wonder about the Freudian "should" and "would." This is another myth — the myth of the so-called "mature" sexuality. According to this myth, the pure, innocent body sensations and curiosities of our childhood have

to be abandoned. The overall sensual pleasures: Rubbing and rocking, poking and stroking, smelling and looking, nuzzling and mouthing — pleasures that aren't yet restricted by any gender rules or genital dominance — have to be given up. I suggest that instead, we had better give up this myth.

We have studied three big myths so far:

MYTH 1 — She should just know.
MYTH 2 — There is no magic if I have to explain.
MYTH 3 — Sex is an instinct that should come naturally.

And now we come upon a fourth:

MYTH 4— Genital sex, meaning vaginal stimulation via penetration, is the only mature sexuality for real women and real men.

Everything else is perverse, childish, regressed, pathetic, and even pathological. We might wonder if such impoverished sex might be a male concept and definition of sexuality. Boys, after all, are taught early on to renounce most or all body pleasure and sensuality. They are not encouraged to give or receive caresses, enjoy bubble baths and body lotions, indulge in a hundred brush strokes through long silky hair, relax in pleasant eternities of being braided all over one's head and fitted with ribbons and pearls, perfumes and powders.

Men's emphasis on purely genital sex, with its focus on penetration, may be the sad outcome of their sensual deprivation in a partriarchal environment. And this culturally enforced, exclusive focus on genital sex may be a way to deprive women,

too. Once a woman is conquered, deflowered, and possessed, our culture's stereotypical sexuality robs her of her sensuous advantages and cripples her natural capacity for overall body involvement and pleasure. Instead of buying into this male model of so-called mature sex, we may decide never to outgrow our childlike sensuality, but instead, to cultivate it.

This is what Sybil and Mariushka chose to do when they went for the polymorphously perverse option. They relearned to play, to "body-play," as they called it. They began to negotiate treats they really wanted, like kids would do: I'll give you this if you give me that. Suddenly, a lot of talk about how these treats should be given led to defining and redefining pleasure.

And yet there was a period when theses pleasures seemed boring to Mariushka, and Sybil complained that this sort of half-innocent body-play clashed with the polyamorous sex fantasies she had learned to cultivate in order to keep up with Mariushka's program. When she understood that there was nothing wrong with any kind of fantasies as long as she was not forcing herself to act on them, they seemed less disturbing to her. Our talking about fantasies created a vivid interest in Mariushka, and the couple introduced "Tell me your dirtiest fantasy" into their sandbox play, which helped Mariushka over her initial boredom. Then it turned into "Tell me your most romantic fantasy," and the fantasies in this new game acquired (in Sybil's words) "terribly sappy story lines." More and more slow, tender, sensuous sensations showed up in the sand-box. Body-play now was mixed with a natural flow of verbal communication, and there even was a hint, and soon more than a hint, of laughing and giggling, burping and farting, and other forbidden regressions.

Mariushka and Sybil reported that they made surprising discoveries about likes and dislikes, in each other and in themselves. In their sandbox, they were permitted to be childish, which meant selfish, greedy, telling the truth about what they wanted or disliked.

The couple often surprised me with their determination to keep the work in the present. The past, their childhood and youth experiences, their parents and family background did not come into the equation for them. The deeper reasons why they had gotten themselves into their impasse, and therefore into the sandbox, did not matter to them. All that mattered was to solve their problem in the here and now — and they were confident all along that they would solve it.

Not everybody wants to make use of analytic insight to make sense of the present through the past. Some people, like Sybil and Mariushka, can work things out through an unfailing enthusiasm for being in the moment, learning to ask for what they want without the need to blame or shame or anxiously protect their vulnerabilities. These two were convinced of their success because of their solid, unchanging attraction to each other. With undiminished zeal, they were now pursuing and acquiring a new, much extended body knowledge and at the same time a language, their own "kid-speak," for their new discoveries. I had promised them early on that they would graduate from the sandbox when they were able to take turns at night stroking each other to sleep.

When I remind them some time later of that goal, Mariushka laughs. "We've decided not to graduate," she declares. "Tell her, hon, what we'll do instead."

Sybil clears her throat. "We want to have sex again, but in

the sandbox, you know? Making love just like that, like kid's play. We want to create a kind of ceremony, a love-sex ceremony to celebrate what we've learned...."

"And we'll end up marrying in the sandbox!" Mariushka slaps her thigh. "Just a joke — marriage would really be the death blow to our sex."

I catch a look from Sybil that seems to say, "Some things will never change."

"Tell me," I ask Mariushka, "what turned it around for you? Is there a moment, a particular event that you recall when Love's Learning Place suddenly didn't seem only ridiculous?"

Mariushka puckers her lips, thinking hard. Then an impish grin appears on her face.

"Remember how I used to shout and holler in the sandbox?" she turns to Sybil. "Because I wanted a quickie, no matter what, no matter how?" She turns back to face me. "I wanted it so badly, I was so fixated on it that I cursed you, I did!" She gives me an apologetic shrug. "But then Sybil said to me one day, 'You don't want your orgasm, it's not even true that you want that! What you want, what you really want, is to have *had* your orgasm, to be done with it. It's not about pleasure, it's not about me or us,' she said to me, 'it's only about your running away from it as fast as you can.' Running away from orgasm.... It's funny, but she was right. I could suddenly see it. All the elaborate games I had invented, with costumes and all, they really allowed me to believe that I was super-super sexual — but I couldn't stand it, in fact...."

"Now you've told it," Sybil says, looking pleased.

"Couldn't stand —?" I invite her to say more.

"Pleasure, I guess."

"Staying with the experience," Sybil adds. "I would very gently stroke her, and she would cry out, I can't stand it, it's too intense, I can't stand it…! And she would want to do something quick and violent to stop it, and to be done."

Mariushka nods. "But Sybil would whisper in my ear, 'You can stand it — I know you, you can't get enough of it!' And that would do it. It was true. I would suddenly surrender, almost collapse, and give up fighting it or controlling it. And then I'd begin to enjoy what she was doing, without wanting anything more, I'd just be there and surrender —" she laughs, "and die, it's such a turn-on!"

She suddenly has the expression of a serious, vulnerable child.

"There's something I never told you," she says. "When I realized that I was just running away from pleasure, I felt so ashamed and desperate at first, and Sybil held me. She just held me in her arms and let me sob. I sobbed a lot. And the way she held me, with no demand, that was…awesome. I think I felt love then, like…you know, like some higher…something. I am not keen on all that spiritual stuff, not normally, but there it was — this new dimension, I don't know.…"

She stops and directs a helpless glance at her lover. Sybil takes her hand, and they look at each other and sigh.

"God, how romantic!" Mariushka can't quite stand it, after all. "But to think that the two of us would do anything romantic.…"

"Just say it, baby," Sybil takes the tone of the Cheshire Cat. "You are a sucker for it. You can't get enough of it, can you?"

Mariushka, to my surprise, blushes. She shrugs, grins, is silent. I think we all know at this moment that there is no need to say more about how much has been accomplished.

In the ending phase of our work together, Sybil and Mariushka pondered at length this new and different, intimate passion that they had discovered in the most unlikely place of their imagination: Their sandbox. Love's Learning Place. They had a hard time believing it but, as we repeatedly found, there was no need to believe it because they were experiencing it, day to day.

Intimate Passion

At this point, we can link the stories of our two couples and draw some conclusions about the role truth plays in uncovering and recovering, kindling and rekindling passion in long-term relationships. When two people together look for truth and tell each other the truth about their bodies, hearts, and minds with tenderness and compassion, role limitations can be transcended, as Lou and Annie discovered, and love can find its passionate expression again. Passion, for Mariushka and Sybil, is no longer a make-believe frenzy that necessarily wears out with repetition, but a consistent radiance that is nurtured through careful, caring attention to what is true at a given moment.

What is this passion that is nourished by the aphrodisiac of truth? And how does it differ from the kind of passion we are used to in our culture?

Passion, as our culture understands it, is the powerful force we have been taught to yearn for. This irresistible force makes us lose our heads in an instant and changes everything that is familiar, to the point that we often don't recognize ourselves any longer. It makes us leave our good old life and partner, burns us with a fire that promises we will be purified, transformed, brought back to life at its most intense and fulfilling. Biochemically speaking, one could compare passion to a supremely potent, natural drug that turns our usual, normal mind-and-body set inside out and upside down. The torment and ecstasy that tend to grip us under the influence of this "drug" are, of course our greatest aphrodisiac, the stuff that our romantic dreams are made of. How does it work, this irresistible force, this sweet violence?

When we look for its ingredients, we find a necessary impersonal element. Passion of this type always relies on distance, on the meeting of strangers, on forbidden and secret yearnings, on fantasies, roles, disguises, rendezvous in exotic places, the risk of the unknown.... This archetypal passion needs obstacles to overcome and resistances to break down. Without obstacles, without resistance, no Passion with a capital P! If the ingredients are right, this fiery Passion has the capacity to overcome cultural inhibitions and physical aversions. Its excitement can break through all defenses and truly sweep us off our feet.

When we get intimate with our passionate lover, however, when the stranger becomes known, when there is no distance any more, when the secret and exotic have given way to the familiar, all our old inhibitions tend to show up again. This is what we experience after the legendary honeymoon: the gradual

retreat back to our normal life, our usual self, our old habits, our old anxieties about being who we always were. With the closeness that comes with getting to know each other in our burdened sexual histories, this great fiery Passion dies.

The not-so-well-known passion, which I call "intimate passion" for contrast, works exactly the other way around: It arises from the intensification of the personal. The only ingredients needed for this intimate passion are a shared attraction and curiosity about who we are in both our most obvious and our most private, secret selves. Intimate passion is a process in which the individual couple works together to undo inhibitions patiently and increasingly, over time. Bodies take time to reveal their secrets, longings, fears, and pleasures. This is what we mean by intimacy — the tender and empathic search for each other with its subtle discoveries and revelations. Intimate passion is nourished by the shared pleasure of knowing how to read each other's mood and erotic body temperature, spelling out each other's alphabet of wishes and desires, knowing in detail and moment by moment how to please and be pleased. With these ingredients, a fundamentally new sexuality awakens. Bodies are grateful creatures: Treat them well, touch them well, and sensual fulfillment will probably be the reward.

The well-known archetypal Passion has its consuming fire and its inevitable end. Intimate passion is a progressive revelation of yet more of the self in a neverending process, which therefore can last until death. Of course, it is possible to pass from the archetypal to the intimate form of passion. Love makes anything possible — truth makes anything possible. For both the couples I have presented, a version of this possibility came into reach. When we evoked this promise in one of our ses-

sions, Annie said wistfully, "Wouldn't it be great to know that you could experience this swoon and bliss after thirty years of marriage with the same partner in bed…?"

It would be great indeed. Just think about it. With enough truth-making, there would be continued lovemaking. With truth as the aphrodisiac, the lovers' bed would no longer be the place of mute misery, faked orgasm, or other lies to get it over with — the place of silent mutiny and refusal; of self-violation in order to overcome disgust; of the mechanical race to orgasm; of boring repetitions of clueless guessing games. With truth's aphrodisiac, the lovers' bed need no longer hold a hundred years of solitude.

If we need a slogan that encapsulates this whole discussion, the one you put on your fridge or on the bathroom mirror, or in embroidery on your favorite pillow, I suggest this one:

"A truth a day keeps the bed death away."

III

Truth as Aphrodisiac

Leap and the net will appear.

— *Julia Cameron*

I magine either of our two couples, or you and your lover. Imagine that this story was told to me, or not. Two women, let's call them Rakisha and Li, are going out for their usual evening walk. They set out shortly before sunset. Rakisha loves the day's last light, Li likes the way the setting sun sees red. They like rituals, these two, and this walk has become a ritual of some sort. It leads past a small pond in a nature area, up a steep path of wooden steps where in spring wild iris grows under the eucalyptus trees. At the top of the stairs, an even smaller path winds along an overhang and into an almost hidden grove of old California oak trees. They have their special tree in the grove, an old oak with a low-set fork of branches easy to step into, the curve of the branch providing just enough room for both of them to sit. Rakisha likes to wrap her arms around the trunk in front of her and tell stories of how, as a young girl, she learned to ride bare-back in the San Cristobal Valley of New Mexico. Li prefers to sit be-

hind her lover and lean comfortably back against the tree trunk. She remembers the horseplay she used to enjoy with her older sister, she the little one, the wild rider who would always be bucked off and tumble to the ground.

"What ground?" Rakisha wants to know.

"Why do you ask?"

"You've told me this story before, but you haven't really told me. I mean, ground? And always with your older sister?"

"Hey, not two questions at the same time. Choose one."

"Ground as in…down pillows, comforter, bedspread?" She wiggles her shoulders evocatively.

Li leans back. "Stop flirting with me. Can't you wait till we get home?"

"You always want to wait. Where's the wild rider now?"

"The wild rider is gonna tumble you off your high horse if you don't watch out." Li gives Rakisha a playful shove with her knee.

Rakisha reaches behind and grabs Li's thighs. "If I tumble, I'll take you down with me." She rocks sideways, pretending to throw both of them off. "To the ground! To the ground! Let's tumble together!"

"Stop rocking. Why can't you sit still?"

Rakisha starts bellowing, "It's now or never, don't hesitate, tomorrow, darling, will be too late!"

"Hush up, pest. You're off key anyway."

"And you've been off all night."

Li puts her hands on Rakisha's shoulders. "Let's not do this, okay? Let's not fight. Let's do what we always like to do."

What these two usually like is to sit in silence and synchronize their breathing. It is their way of entering nature and each

other's thoughts. They often stay until it's almost dark or the frogs over at the little pond begin croaking.

"Okay, let's try," Rakisha says, but after ten seconds she kicks out her legs, throws her arms out above her head and shouts, "Yippeee...!"

"What is it with you today?" Li grabs her wrists and holds them down against her thighs.

Rakisha starts rocking back and forth against her lover's body. "Ride with me, come on, ride with me. Or else tell me about your so-called sister...."

"I'll tell you if you promise to be good."

"I'll be good." Rakisha inches toward Li. "Very, very, very good."

Li is pensive, rubs her cheek against her lover's face. "It's true, one time ..."

"One time? One time? What happened one time?"

"Hush. Listen. You wanted to know about the ground, remember?"

"I'm listening."

"So, there was this sheepskin in front of my sister's bed. There was the prickly grass of the neighborhood park. There was the sand at that island we used to visit in the summer, where my uncle had his summer house and our whole family could vacation free of charge, which meant a lot to us then because..."

"Yes, yes, yes. We know that story."

"You think you know that story."

"I don't?"

"Nobody knows that story."

"Not even your sister?"

"Never mind my sister...."

"Well? Go on...."

Li hesitates. "I don't really feel like going into all that right now. Let's just be silent, that always works for us."

"Maybe it always works for you."

"But it's good for you, you know it yourself. It's always better when you calm down, you've said it a thousand times...."

"You've said it a thousand times and I've agreed."

"Don't you agree?"

"Are you going to tell your story or not?"

"I told you, I'm not in the mood."

"Yes, you are. I know you, you're just hedging. That story, I need to hear it. Come on baby, give it to me." She reaches for Li's hand.

"Come on baby, come on baby...I've heard that before."

"Somebody had to coax you? How come? You're always the one who says, 'Shut up, do this, do that, do it my way.'"

"Are you saying..." Li withdraws her hand.

"Yes, you are controlling. You've been in a controlling mood all night, trying to stop me, and I'm really beginning to wonder why."

"Come on. We're out in public and you're shouting and kicking your legs and singing every kind of nonsense...."

"Public?" Rakisha looks around dramatically. "You mean the skunks and the deer and the owl are going to overhear us?"

"You know what I mean. If I didn't hold you back sometimes, you know what would happen."

"Yeah, if you wouldn't hold me back sometimes I would do something to you that you might enjoy too much, eh?"

"You're getting very personal. I don't like it."

"Go ahead. Control that too. Control me all the way, so there's no danger left." Rakisha suddenly flings her leg over the branch, swivels around and faces Li. "You are scared of something. If only you would tell me what."

Li squints at her. "And now you're trying to control me in return? And make me?"

"Yes, I want to make you. Yes, I do. I want to make you." She takes her lover's face in both her hands. "But I don't want to make you afraid."

Li has closed her eyes. "It would be too good to be true."

"If I made you, you mean?"

"I hate that language." Li turns her face away. "You make someone do something and then you think you made them? But you can't make me because..."

"Was that what happened?" Rakisha is suddenly still.

Li looks taken by surprise. "Maybe —"

 "And it wasn't with your sister?"

Li searches her lover's eyes. "There were always lots of kids around. We played lots of games in the dunes and on the beach."

"Yeah, and? And?" Rakisha shoves her face close and shakes Li lightly by her shoulders.

"You really want to hear this?"

"Yes, honey. Dear one. I really, really want it."

Li takes a deep breath. "That day, my sister was supposed to baby-sit me. But she ran away with some older kids. She left me with another little girl, a real bossy little thing from the bungalow next door. Katie. Who had already taught me to pick my nose."

"You? Picking your nose?"

"Well, it had never occurred to me."

"O honey…"

"It just never had. Anyway, my sister ran off with the others, and she ordered us to stay put in that hollow in the dunes. Katie said, 'Let's bury you.' I loved being buried. I remember it seemed to take a long time. Katie was heaping and dribbling the hot sand over my legs, first my feet, then my knees, then piling it all around me until I was completely covered. I think I must have slumped back and closed my eyes. It felt so good, the sand running and tickling my skin. Then Katie shrieked, 'You're all gone, where are you, where are you, you're all gone.' I sat up. She said, 'Let's try to find you,' digging for my belly. I tried to say, 'I'm right here,' and Katie said, 'Where are you, let's try to find you.' I was mesmerized. She stuck her hands into the sand and touched my legs. 'You're not there,' she said, pulling her hands out and sticking them in again, closer to my bathing suit…you know where. Only the thing was, I didn't know where that was, or what that was…."

"You didn't know where that was?"

"Damn right. I was only five and my mother was always after me. I mean, if you're not allowed to pick your nose. I mean, if you haven't even figured out that you could pick your own nose. And your older sister doesn't know either…."

"Wow. Five years old. But I knew. I found out riding those horses…"

"What do you mean? I was riding my sister and I didn't find out anything."

"Well, I guess that's what happens when you grow up in the Basin. But in the country…"

"So what did you find out? I mean, how did you find it out riding a horse? I mean, did somebody show you?"

"Are you kidding? Show me? Honey, did you ever ride bare-back on a horse? If the horse is cantering and you want to hold on you have to squeeze your legs, you know. So there's this rhythm, and this riding, the horse's backbone, and this squeezing. You get it?"

"I guess a horse is a better teacher than a sister."

"Anyway, this isn't about me. Somehow or other you did find out. What did you find out?"

"All I knew was that Katie's hand was down there doing ... I don't know exactly what. And down there was just not a down there I'd ever come across, not like that. My mother was pretty rough when she washed me. But this was inde-scribable, a sweetness that put me in a complete swoon. I wanted this to go on forever and ever. Seeing nothing, hearing noth-ing, saying nothing — just swoon on and on. Forever. Until this loud shriek came. My sister's voice, I think it was my sister, brought me back. It was horrible, absolutely horrible, there they stood, all those older kids, pointing at us, and Katie thought it was really funny. She jumped up and joined the others, laughing her head off, while I just sat there in the sand, still out of it...."

"My god, that's terrible. God, that's awful. Had they planned that?"

"Of course not. I don't know. I don't think so. I mean, could they have planned that? With Katie? Not my sister. Never. She knew less than I did...."

"Oh honey, even if they didn't plan it, I still want to wring their necks!"

"But that's not the worst. One of the kids, a really mean boy, shouted back at me, while they were all running away, and

Katie with them, 'We'll tell your parents, we'll tell everyone!' I was terrified. I had no idea what I had done. Or, well, somehow I knew this was so awful I wanted to die. But I liked it. That was the worst of it. I wanted to die because of that too. Because I couldn't stop feeling it. That sweetness."

"O yes, that sweetness. Thank God you never stopped feeling it."

"But I did, all of a sudden I did. I didn't feel it any more, and I never felt it again. Not really. At least, not until I moved away from home to go to college."

Rakisha throws her arms around her lover. "Oh honey, those damn kids. I can't believe it." She strokes Li's hair out of her face and scrutinizes her. "So it got buried under the sand. For all those years. That's hard to imagine. Because I kept on all those years just riding horses."

"But that's something you were doing by yourself. It didn't involve other people."

"Well, after a while it involved other people...."

"You never told me that part."

"Sure I did, I told you how I started already at eleven."

"True, you told me that. I don't like to think about it because I sometimes envy you. I never truly reconnected with that sweetness. Not really, really. I realize that now. I never went back to that moment as a child."

"Not even with me? Really? Do you mean that?"

"Maybe for moments. Moments."

"Moments when you feel like that little five-year-old girl again?"

"I really never made the connection before. It seems so obvious but somehow it escaped me. There are those funny moments

when I would like time to stand still, to go into that sort of swoon and be completely...you know."

"Under the sand?"

"Yes, like that time...."

"Passive?"

Li hides her face again against Rakisha's shoulder. "A late confession," she says in a small voice.

It's dark and neither of them has noticed. Usually they are already on their way home, but not tonight. Rakisha is stroking Li's head and neck. Stroking her shoulders. Her back. "These moments," she says, into her lover's ear, "what do I do when they happen? Tell me. No, come on, tell me."

"You do...I don't know how to tell. You do something but you do almost nothing."

"You mean, I have my hand like this..."

"You have your hand there."

"I move a little?"

"Just a little."

"Like I am trying to find you?"

"Trying to ..."

"Find you out?"

"Find me out."

"Like this?"

"Like this.

"You mean, like Katie?"

"Like Katie. Yes, yes, like that, like Katie...."

IV

TRUE CONFESSIONS

Approach love and cooking with reckless abandon.

— *H.H., the 14th Dalai Lama*

The Icing on the Cake

At our first meeting, I learn that Selena is a forty-some-thing Mexican-American and Petra a forty-year-old from "Midwestern solid German stock." There is something solid indeed about my first impression of them. Both are large, beautiful women exuding calm and friendly balance. Selena has long dark curls, Petra a straight blond mane down to her shoulders. They choose the sofa, holding hands, and both give me a long, expectant smile.

"What brings you in?" I inquire.

They look at each other and back at me. "We don't really know why we're here," Selena finally says. "We shouldn't be here, but…"

"Selena thinks we have a problem," Petra says.

"Not a problem-problem," Selena says reassuringly. "It's just that Petra has a question."

"Not really," Petra says. "Selena just thinks I'm not happy."

"Do you have an idea why Selena thinks that?" I ask.

"Selena thinks I should..." she squeezes Selena's hand to make her talk.

"Not true!" Selena blurts out. They burst into laughter.

"That's the problem, " Selena explains, "we are too happy in a way. We aren't normal."

Petra leans back and sighs.

I inquire what is not normal about being happy.

Petra strokes a curl from Selena's cheek. "When I met Selena at a women's fund raiser for Salvadorian refugees, I was right away attracted. By her power. She is a great talker. We have a very similar view of social politics, and we found that we liked each other's ideas and ideals. And afterwards, we danced together and that did it, I think. There was such synchronicity in our dancing, our rhythm, our energy..."

"...and sensuality," Selena nods with a big smile. "Yes, love at first sight and at first dance."

"Selena ended up moving to Oakland and doing fund-raising for some of the women's projects I am involved in. We're a great team working together, always inspired by each other. A good two years ago, we moved in together with another couple, forming a collective, you know. Now we're a couple and part of a collective, and part of a group of women makers and shakers. It's wonderful, just what we always dreamed of." They beam at each other.

"It sounds very happy indeed," I comment. "Where's the too happy? What's not normal?"

Again Petra answers, "It's in our private life. We spend a lot of time together. At home, whenever we can. On the couch, in the tub, on the sofa.... Our roommates think this is great, that

the world would be a better place if everybody would be loving like this. We think so too, don't we?" She turns to Selena. "But the other day our friend Lakeisha came in with a survey on sex, and she wanted to know things about our sex life, how often we did it and all that...."

"She asked us how often we come when we make love," Selena sounds embarrassed. "It kind of threw us."

There is a long silence.

"We don't come, we're always there but we don't come," Selena continues. "That's not normal, is it?" she asks me.

Before I can answer Petra shakes her head. "I so disagree with 'not normal,'" she says, raising her voice for the first time. "My volleyball coach always used to say, 'Normal is ninety-seven degrees, that's what normal is!'"

"I don't understand. Explain it to me," I say.

Petra passionately describes a love life made of cuddling, tenderness, long sessions of hugging, kissing, rolling around, giggling, talking, gazing. Selena follows the description with appreciative smiles and nods. I get the picture of a sensuality that is equally shared and intensely satisfying for both. Petra sums it up: "Isn't this everyone's dream? We sleep completely rolled up in each other. We nap like that."

"We even do yoga like that," Selena jokes. "But we never have sex."

"Not true," Petra blushes and her voice goes up several notches. "This is just the same old political bullshit. We are so sexy and so sexual in all our doings, why shouldn't that count as sex?"

"Who's counting?" I ask.

"Exactly," Petra nods, "Selena counts."

"I don't count," Selena says, "there's nothing to be counted."

"Nothing!" Petra sounds really hurt.

"Say more," I address Selena.

"When Lakeisha came with her survey I was embarrassed. I suddenly felt it wasn't all that great. I mean, no orgasms, no sex, what is it that we are doing?" Selena looks at Petra, who looks close to tears.

"Why does it always have to go further?" Petra says, plaintively. "Why isn't it enough to be held and caressed all over, kissed everywhere...?"

"Everywhere?" I ask.

Selena seems unsure while Petra insists, "Everywhere. Even down there. Nothing is left out. Nothing."

"Except orgasm," Selena shrugs.

At the end of our first session I am puzzled. My first thought goes to wondering if there is any history of sexual abuse. Any physical or emotional trauma? Are the two of them presenting me with the truth? In the following sessions we establish that there is indeed no obvious reason for any limitation to their intimacy. When I take their sexual histories I learn that while Selena has had orgasmic relationships and occasionally masturbates to orgasm, Petra never does.

Petra made a few teenaged attempts at dating, but never went beyond petting. She was seventeen when she decided she wasn't interested in boys. She liked girls much better. Shortly afterwards, she discovered feminism, and developed a firm political conviction that the absence of sexual arousal and orgasm was the desirable corrective to the dominant, male-dominated sexual attitudes of our society. She wasn't abstinent, she tells me, she was simply fed up with the "screw-obsession that hangs over our heads day and night." She was proud to be a "full-bred

political lesbian," which, in her eyes, was so much more than "just following the dictates of what men call nature."

"I got so mad when I saw that survey," she says. "Not that there was anything new there. It's always the same. 'How often do you have sex?' Meaning: Men's sex! Penetration! Nothing else is counted. Men can have it every day, several times a day. Women? Nobody asks us, not really. Women don't tell the truth in these surveys. But the minute they are alone with their girlfriends, you hear it. They can do without it. Men get it up, get on top, get off, get off on it. And then they have their great day in the surveys. Men have so much sex! But the women — all the women I've talked to want what we have, Selena and I. They are starved for tenderness and for touching. Once you have a woman by herself, and a glass of wine, you hear the true story. All they get is *Wham, bam, thank you, Ma'm.* That's what sex is. I refuse to have any part in that. Fuck this society. We need another sexual revolution, if you ask me. Selena and I have made a start."

When Petra goes into her political sex discourse, Selena's expression changes from proud to somewhat doubtful.

When I ask Selena about her take on all of this, she says that on the whole she is very comfortable with Petra's views. She describes coming from a family of powerful Yucatan women where good eating, lots of touching, sensuality and beauty and heated family discussions — led by the women — were part of everyday life.

"When I took Petra to my family, even though she didn't speak Spanish at first, she just fit right in and seemed to understand everything that was going on like another sister. So who am I to complain that this happiness is missing out on

one little detail? If it's all that important to me, I can give it to myself. Although I know Petra is critical of this kind of patriarchal sensation-seeking…"

"…this damned conditioning of Western culture," Petra says loudly. "To climax rather than enjoy. Why should one end pleasure? Just because men can't sustain it…."

"Well, does it really have to end there?" Selena looks at me for support. "I am not so sure any more. It is, after all, part of my culture…."

"What is?" Petra asks.

"Getting hot, turning the heat up, chili stuff, you know…."

"Don't say we are not having that…."

"Honestly," Selena looks nervously at me, "I think we really don't. But if we wanted even more, wouldn't it be like male greed, at least in Petra's eyes? I mean, whenever we get close to the real salsa, Petra is blissfully falling asleep."

Petra stands up, grabs her bag and says, "This is not going anywhere. If you want to complain in here I'm out of it. If that is all you have to say about me, that I'm falling asleep like a … a head of cabbage or something, it's not worth spending money here."

She stops in her tracks, looks embarrassed, looks at Selena, drops her bag. "Okay, okay," she says turning to me, "I didn't mean it. Sorry, Renate, it's really not about money."

"What's it about?" I ask, while she sits down again. "What's wrong with falling asleep?"

Petra invites Selena with a sweeping gesture. "Go ahead, tell the dirty truth."

Selena humphs, seemingly unruffled by Petra's temper tantrum. "Dirty, all right. I have to say I've never really understood

what is so intolerable to Petra about orgasm. Or, in fact, even just excitement. I know she doesn't like it and I have stopped trying to convince her that it could also be nice."

"Nice?" I ask. "Is that all it is?"

She raises her eyebrows. "Noooo…but I guess I have convinced myself to be just as happy without it. Maybe it would spoil everything…for Petra or, I mean, between us.…Then we would be like everybody else, wouldn't we? Always chasing after this one thing. Like with eating, if you always leave yourself a little appetite the next taste is so much the better, isn't it?"

"You never eat to your heart's content?"

They both laugh. I see their glances sweeping over each other's luscious, full-breasted bodies.

Petra says, "We can't hide that. Eating is better than sex, if you ask me."

Selena purrs: "I sometimes wish I could eat you all up and just go out of my mind.…"

Petra gasps. "What would be left of me?" she asks in the voice of a little girl.

"A puddle of pleasure," Selena says.

Petra's whole body withdraws into her corner of the couch. Her anxious, pleading face tells us some hidden truth has been touched and desperately wants to stay in hiding.

Petra and Selena raise a significant issue. Women's inclination for an all-over body sensuality can certainly be seen as an immense gift of nature. Many women, especially women who have lived with and been sexual with men, find extraordinary delight in discovering the sensual dimension in their love relationship with a woman. So many complain that their men were never interested in more than the three erotic zones of

their bodies — mouth, breasts, and genitals; that their diet of body delights was decidedly anorexic. Now they luxuriate in a twelve-course meal with their woman lover, rediscovering that their bodies are covered all over in skin, and that skin relishes so many different kinds of contact and touch. Indeed, like Petra, they feel they have discovered a world unknown to heterosexual society and are fiercely proud, even militant, about their revelation of the female body's capacity for pleasure. The genital predominance of our heterosexual society's approach to sex is understandably criticized by many of these women, but it is still not clear why some of them, like Petra, wish to exclude orgasmic sex altogether.

Petra would insist that her exclusion of "intercourse" is a purely political choice. In my work with Petra and Selena, it turned out to have psychological meaning as well. When we explored her growing up, we found that Petra's surroundings were dominated by an excitable, volatile father who had only recently been diagnosed as manic-depressive. The mother, a very strong, Germanic woman, pretended to be the captain of their family ship. She always found a positive, optimistic explanation for everything the father did, including the sale of their family home while she and the children were on vacation. With every promising new job the father took on, the family was dragged to a new place. The shifts from wealth to poverty overnight left the mother exhausted and bereft, but still fiercely maintaining that her husband was the greatest dad. Petra grew up hating any excitement, any intense stimulation, any exultation. The ideal of her young years was equanimity, harmony, and balance. Orgasms would have upset this program.

In one of our sessions, she was able to narrate an unsettling

experience she had when she was fifteen years old.

"We were off for a weekend with our championship volley-ball team. I was rooming with Susie. Susie was what we today would call cool. I totally admired her, because she was more in control than anyone on our team. She moved like a panther, never broke into a sweat, and yet was the fastest of us all. No one could return her serve, I mean no one.

When she made a move on me I was so floored that for a while I was convinced everything she was doing could only be just right. You know how I figured out that something was going on? When I came back into our room after taking a shower I saw that she had moved our two beds together. She pounced on me, grabbed me in a bear hug, tumbled me on the bed until we both fell on the floor. She pinned me down and kissed me and I completely lost it...."

Selena has been looking at her like she has never seen her before. "Lost it? Lost what? What do you mean, lost it?"

"I didn't know what to do. My head was spinning, I didn't know where up was and what was down, there were her hands all over me and then even her... I had no idea what she was doing down there, I was trying to pull her by her hair but she only laughed and grabbed my wrists and went on...."

I motion to Selena to sit back in her chair and not interrupt her.

Petra looks petrified. "It was terrible, somehow, but I couldn't stop it, I didn't know how to stop it." She suddenly waves her arms like a windmill, as if to alleviate a hot flash. "Pooh," she shouts, "I don't want to remember this."

Selena leans over to put both arms around her shoulders, "Please honey, don't be scared, go on, this is it...."

Petra moves out of the embrace, covers her face with her hands, leaning forward to put her elbows on her knees. She is breathing heavily. She shakes her head, as if to indicate she can't go on. In a muffled voice, she brings out, "I thought I was having a heart attack, my heart was going so fast and my breath too, I couldn't get air, I even began shaking, my legs kept shaking, she was rocking me ... something so hot I thought I was burning ... I screamed, I heard myself scream, that stopped her. It was a rape, it was a rape...."

"It wasn't a rape, honey, " Selena says, "it was an orgasm! It can feel like that the first time...."

Petra is stunned. She lifts her head and looks completely bewildered. "Are you kidding? An orgasm? You mean I had ..." Her voice dies.

"It sure sounds like that," Selena almost chuckles.

"Whatever it was, Petra," I say, "it must have been very frightening. What you are describing sounds as if you suddenly had lost your usual control over your body. That's when you felt you had lost it. When the excitement of arousal happens all at once, without a warning, without any slow preparation and buildup of desire, it can feel like violence."

Selena says, "Honey, you had an orgasm. You had an orgasm."

Petra glares at her. "Yeah. Okay. And I'll tell you what. I will never let anyone put me through that again."

Selena puts her arms back around Petra. "Don't you worry, sweetheart. Nobody will put you through that again. Next time, you'll be in control, and that'll make all the difference."

Explorer in an Unknown Land

Needless to say, Petra resisted this oracular reassurance by her lover. But after many conversations, Petra began to understand two things: How deeply Selena wished for their bond to grow and become sexually exciting as well as sensually fulfilling; and that her extreme fear of excitement had its origin in her father's disturbing manic episodes. If she continued to avoid excitement in any intimate form, she remained the victim of her father. This idea of being Daddy's girl against her will was outrageous enough for Petra to want to take action. Her feminist optimism became a great help in taking the bull by the horns and challenging her early family conditioning. She designed her own new program of sexual liberation, refusing suggestions from me and even from Selena. She was determined to have everything under her very own control.

Petra could not imagine at first that an orgasm could be approached and experienced in a gradual, gentle, incremental fashion — in short, that it could be learned like any other bodily experience. But Petra was able to articulate what many women find mysterious about their sexual experience: She could narrate from within the difficulties of sexual arousal. She often insisted how frightening the entire experience was, that something was taking her over and she didn't know what it was, where it began, where it would go, if it would ever stop. She didn't like the idea of somebody else playing her body like an instrument. She was scared of being at somebody's

mercy. What if the excitement began, what if she felt desire for being touched, more and more, and the other person suddenly stopped and refused to let her go on? What if her body wanted it so badly she'd do anything to get it? Would she be judged as a needy, greedy monster? A nymphomaniac? What if she got used to it and couldn't do without it, and the other person wasn't around any more?

These are some of the fears many women have to contend with, especially before they have gathered bodily and sexual experience, and no wonder. Who is it that speaks frankly with girls about this powerful event of the body? Doesn't our culture assume that sex is so natural, so instinctual, that sexual pleasure must be likewise? One can't ask often enough: Do we have a language, even if we wanted to talk about it? A language specific, precise, and yet subtle enough to capture the physical sensation, the arousal, the transformation of the body into the sexual body — the body of desire — wishing for and demanding its own pleasure and fulfillment? Without any help, without guidance, without language, so many women find themselves limping through this glorious landscape with a body crippled in one way or another by fear, shame, overwhelm, ignorance.

Petra was lucky. Selena was accustomed to gentleness and patience and therefore was able to move at Petra's pace, without taking one step ahead of Petra herself. Petra took courage from the fact that she, herself, brought some knowledge to the difficult task of learning sexual excitement and surrender. She already knew a vast repertoire of body pleasures. She had fair precision in knowing and communicating what felt good and what didn't. My suggestion that she learn to masturbate didn't fly. The idea of facing the dangers all alone, by herself,

was too much. She wanted Selena there to reassure and comfort her, and at the same time to arouse her. She scheduled special weekend times with Selena to venture out into her sexual territory. She told me she felt like her German ancestors when they set out as pioneers, entering a dangerous but alluring unknown land. The idea itself began to excite her, and at some point she asked for a small break in therapy to be "on her own" like a real explorer. But orgasm, as she reported in short weekly e-mail messages, continued to elude her.

This is a familiar stage of learning: After an initial enthusiasm and exciting start we tend to hit a snag and feel stuck again, or we come to a plateau where some progress shows, but our ultimate goal is still out of reach.

After a couple of months at that stage, Petra and Selena come in with long faces, declaring, "It's not working. It's never going to work. We have decided to go back to where we've come from. We've had it so good — why all this fuss to make it even better? Isn't there a kind of proverbial saying, 'Leave well enough alone?'"

I ask them to explain.

Selena says: "It makes both of us unhappy. I'm working on Petra's orgasm, I'm jumpy and agitated because I get overexcited and I don't know what to do with it. I want to grab her and eat her up, but mostly I just want to shake her!" She notices Petra's anxious face and adds, "Oh honey, don't look like that. I don't mean it."

Petra sounds defeated: "It's like climbing Mount Everest. You never get beyond base camp. And what's it for? Why climb to the top if the view from here is pretty neat? It's satisfying, has always been."

I say, "What is sexuality for? That is a good question."

Selena says impatiently, "Well, we don't know any more. You tell us."

Petra elbows her: "It's not *her* fault."

"I understand that you are frustrated," I say. "You had a vision of something and now it sounds like you simply want to give up halfway. You sound irritated. It's like you show a child a chocolate cake and then only give it a crumb. You may feel like that about me right now. But what about the chocolate cake that has been right here in front of you? On your mind, in your imagination — you saw it, didn't you? Where's it now?"

Selena sighs. "You're right. Now we pretend it's only a crumb and we can forget about it...."

"I don't think I ever knew what's the big deal about that cake," Petra says. "Could someone please explain it to me again?"

"Come on now," Selena smiles, "you know. All the things we always do. That's the cake, and then there's the icing, which we haven't had. And some people, well many people, think the icing is the best part of the cake."

"Do you?" I ask.

"I guess so. I honestly have a hard time seeing how I could be without it."

"What do you mean by icing?" I ask.

"O, I don't mean just orgasm. I mean a really exciting sexual tension, all that hot stuff, that chili stuff," she repeats.

"You must be crazy," Petra protests, "to think our beautiful cake is nothing without that stupid icing."

Why Have Sex?

Petra and Selena are expressing what many couples feel after the sexual excitement has quieted down and maybe even
disappeared from the relationship altogether. It doesn't seem
to matter that Petra and Selena have come to this predicament without ever having experienced this excitement together.
At this point they are like all other couples who don't have it
and wonder if it's worth working and pining for.

In my opinion, this fundamental question has not been asked
enough: What purpose is served by sex? Why is it so necessary
to go on having sex at the age of fifty, sixty, seventy... or after
ten years of a relationship? Why is it always in tragic tones
that couples report, "We haven't had sex in two months!" although they have been affectionate with each other during that
time? It is remarkable how many times I have heard that question, "Why have sex?" — posed rhetorically — from women
who feel they are so close, so intimate that they believe they
could not be closer. Isn't it good enough to have the physical
comfort, soothing, tenderness that women so easily develop with
each other? Is it just another patriarchal myth that they should
have more action in their beds? Their closeness is already far
beyond any intimacy they think the sex act could achieve. I
would argue that the quality of closeness that comes through
a fulfilling sexual relationship has profoundly different elements
than does any other closeness. Sexual surrender, the risk of it,
the implied trust involved in giving up control to a beloved

other, brings about a quality of deep emotion that can only be experienced in the body, where body and heart and soul and spirit beat together in the same rhythm.

Wilhelm Reich was probably right on in his claim that a truly fulfilling orgasm has benefits for the entire energy system of the body — for physical and emotional balance and health. But there is much more to it, in my view.

When we are intensely fond of another person we often find ourselves, as Selena did, experiencing the nervous tension of over-stimulated children who don't know what to do with themselves. We feel we are going insane with desire; we can't stand the deluge of feeling. We want to squeeze the adored body and tear it to pieces like delicious dough, bite big chunks out of it, incorporate it, devour it whole, and be done with it. These are powerful and even violent feelings, and there literally seems to be no channel for these primal desires apart from making love. In the absence of sexual expression, this buildup of tension has to be bottled up, held back, put to sleep. Or it may be discharged in anger, irritation, a fight — attempts to turn this unsettling tension down some familiar road. Indeed, if these powerful energies don't find appropriate expression, they can become destructive and self-destructive. Love is a strange, hungry beast. If we don't feed it, it turns against us. Our frustration, anger, irritation, and confusion can become so intense that we are compelled outside our long-term couple to an ex-lover, a friend wishing to experiment with woman-to-woman sex, or a one-night stand with a stranger encountered at a woman's bookstore.

But if we face the beast, if we cultivate the innate knowledge that Love's Learning Place has revealed, there is a reward. Our couple is constantly renewed through the primordial depths to

which sex gives access. In the moments of letting go, forgetting ourselves completely in the safe embrace, reawakening in the arms of our lover, we can enter a place of rebirth. Sex allows a couple to be bathed in primordial waters. The transformative power of the experience tends to be felt all through the body, through all the senses, in a way that opens us up to the greater powers of nature and the universe — the Goddess, the divine. We take part in something inexplicable, larger and more powerful than our minds, so that for many women orgasm in this sense has a profoundly spiritual and unifying meaning. Some women speak about this spiritual dimension of lovemaking, the free and complete circulation of energy through every chakra, as the "orgasm of the heart." There are some who achieve it through the gaze alone, the meeting of souls between lovers; but this orgasm, too, requires risk, encounter, trust, active desire, and surrender. It requires the same capacity to take as to give, to be fully in the moment, to be undefended, in order that we may meet the other in the unknown.

When we discuss this quality of physical/sexual love in our session, Petra and Selena have no problem recognizing the difference between their cozy, risk-free nesting and this high-risk adventure with the icing on the cake. They decide to continue their journey across the unknown continent.

Soon, there is a surprise. Halfway through the session, I learn that Petra's growing capacity for desire and excitement is suddenly not met by a similar arousal in Selena.

"I don't understand," Petra says. "I really get off but now Selena dozes off. She won't respond."

"Are you saying you have changed roles? You are not falling asleep anymore, Petra? But Selena is?"

Big smile from Selena. "Well, truth is, we've always fallen asleep together, haven't we? Now I can't stop. Sex has been our symbiotic sleeping pill. I think I get tired working Petra up to orgasm."

"Or could it be that you get overexcited too soon and you've found your way back to your familiar way of turning that off?"

"Yeah, exactly. That's it."

"You two. I'm always impressed by your readiness to tell the truth without much ado. But go on. There must be more. Working people up to orgasm? It doesn't sound very hot to me either. Work and pleasure, work and play … you know what I think about that."

Selena says, "Okay, it's that I seem to always hit a wall with Petra. She gets so happy, so aroused, totally wet, I can tell she wants it, I know she wants more, she wants to come and I simply can't understand why she doesn't. She won't let go."

Petra shakes her head. "I sure want to. But you just won't get me over the edge. I keep telling you what to do…."

"No way, you're not communicating clearly. And frankly. Don't make it my fault. I do everything you want me to…."

I stop them. "Perhaps something is wanted by both of you that has not yet been said — perhaps has not even been found. It must be very difficult for you, Selena, to be so unsuccessful."

Selena chokes up. "But is it me? Am I being unsuccessful? It often really makes me mad. Really mad. I want to shake her out of it, or into it…I don't know. She is walling me off, she just won't go on, it feels like she's slamming a door on me, or refusing to open one. I feel so alone and left out and meanwhile she's blaming me. It's my fault, I'm not doing it right,

I'm not touching her right, ever. That can't be."

Petra says, "Okay, maybe you're right. But it really feels like you're never understanding me. I wish I could...I could..."

"Petra," I say, "in your wildest dreams, if you had a magic spell over the bed — what would happen? Dream it up, tell us what you wish for. Really wish for. Tell us the secret."

Petra blushes. "No way. I could never. Not tell. I would die of shame. It's too ... ridiculous. What I sometimes wish for is so not PC [politically correct]. No, no, I'd rather die."

"Hello!" Selena shouts. "I knew it. I just knew it. A dirty secret after all. O honey, this is too good. Tell, tell, try, give a hint, I'll guess the rest."

"Stop it, stop it, don't push, don't...rape me...." Petra's voice is rising. She flashes me a glance that says, "Save me. Get her off me...!"

I end the session and send them home for a big hug. I tell them they have accomplished a decisive step in their closeness. The existence of a secret has been revealed, although the secret itself has not yet been told. I trust that the two of them will find it out in their private time and space. I know them by now, and I am sure Petra will not end up feeling raped by Selena's eagerness to know her.

In our next session, Petra says: "I don't know what's going on with me. I want to be held by Selena, but not just held. Held, I mean, as if I were just a little thing. And I don't fit with my big body, I mean this is ridiculous, I, a little thing with this ...look at me...huge. I feel so silly, but for some reason I can't laugh about it. Or maybe I can, but if *she* does I get awfully hurt. I want her to take it seriously no matter how silly it is, but it is silly, isn't it? I can't take it seriously myself."

Selena interprets, "I get the feeling that Petra really wants to feel like an infant or something. And be held by me like a mother would hold a..."

"But I've always felt that we were mothering each other," Petra interrupts. "And that's always been fine, why isn't it now?"

Selena says, "Because it's not equal now, that's why."

I encourage her to say more.

She hesitates. "I feel a real shift here. Petra wants me not just to be motherly but to baby her in a real sense. I don't know how to explain.... Why does it matter which way I hold her?"

Petra is puzzled. "I wish I knew. There is just such a special feeling when I lie at your breast in that way. It makes me cry, it makes me...I can't even tell what it makes me... it just does." She has tears in her eyes. "I need you to understand. I just goddamn need you to understand and do it right."

Selena says: "But it can't be done right. You're so picky. You used to like everything but now you're becoming too specific for me, I can't keep up with you, you're demanding and insistent and I feel like a failure. It makes me mad. You're bossing me around like a...like a baby brat. I get the impression if babies could talk, they'd be demanding things just like you...."

"It makes me mad too, if you want to know. There you suddenly come with a judgment. I think what you can't stand in fact is that I really want this. That I need it. That you are really needed, for once."

I intervene. "Selena wasn't needed before?"

There is a pause. Petra looks on the verge of crying.

"This is different. It's so needy-needy, there's no word for it, really. It's like I am really just being born and my life depends on it, getting it. I'm so naked and little and desperate...." She

covers her face with her hands.

Selena strokes her. "It's all right, honey. I want to hear it. I'm not making judgments. I need to hear it...."

Petra whispers, "I'm in danger. It's dangerous there. What if you really do what I want and I really get what I want and then you suddenly don't...what then? What would I do then?"

Selena looks at me with questioning eyes. "You mean, the minute you are getting close you are afraid it's gonna be taken away? You haven't even got there yet and you are already so scared that I'll do something to stop you?"

I say, "Hold it, Selena. There's a step missing. Wanting something is a vulnerable thing. If we can experience wanting and having a wish fulfilled, then we are learning at the same time that the fulfillment could also be withheld."

Selena says, "But I would never."

"It's a leap of faith," I say. "The first time you have to jump to know that your lover will catch you. How else could you build up trust?"

"Trust it, trust me," Selena urges. "I'll catch you."

"It's not that easy," Petra protests. She lowers her hands from her face just enough to glower at me, then hides again. "I *am* embarrassed," she murmurs through her hands. "I feel I'm humiliating myself... maybe.... If I'm really such a baby, how can I maintain my power in this relationship? At the next fight, it might come up against me in a *big* way."

"You're afraid that Selena could humiliate and ridicule you because she knows what you need and want so much?" I ask.

"But it's what both of us want so much," Selena protests. "Have I ever done that to you? I never would and you know it...."

"You might not know you want it, but maybe you want it just because I want it...."

"Want what?" Selena demands.

"I'd become your thing, your slave or something." Petra now hides behind her arms as if to protect herself from a beating. "You know what I want, I want it so badly I'd do anything to get it and still it always depends on you and you can decide." She sounds miserable, while Selena listens, looking increasingly alarmed. "My entire pleasure depends on you, there's nothing equal any more," Petra goes on lamenting. "Everything we had is destroyed because now...now you have the power and I don't...."

Selena throws her curls back in anger. "Give me a break, hon. Stop your PC rants about equality. If equality was really that sexy you would have orgasms every five minutes, every day ...." She rolls her eyes around as if she can't believe she has just said this.

Petra comes up from behind her arms. She looks stunned.

I say, "Let's not forget that equality is the foundation of your relationship and cannot that easily be shaken by difference. If you let Selena have the power to fulfill your wishes, Petra, who says you won't have the same power to fulfill hers?"

They both stare at me as if I had just fired a shot.

"You mean Selena's going to have to go through this too?" Petra doesn't sound miserable any more.

"No way," Selena shrieks, letting her hair fall over her face.

"Hach, Renate says, you too!" Petra shouts triumphantly, checking in with me that she's on the right track. "Fair is fair."

Selena produces a belly laugh that Petra happily joins.

"Wait, just wait," Petra says, "ve haf vays to mak you."

"Mature Sex"

Wishes, especially bodily wishes, can lead us straight back into childhood experiences and thus bring back the powerful experience of being the victim of overpowering needs, hungers, sensations. Wishes make us reexperience the tensions of the child's helplessness and impotence that depend, for release, on the presence of an all-powerful mother. Sex, in blatant disregard of our so-called "genital maturity," constantly throws us back into the pool of those primal sensations. Indeed, as I have pointed out before, the whole notion of "genital maturity" is just another myth, a fantasy that aims to free us from the child's original body experience. Wouldn't it be the perfect easy way out, the perfect evasion, if this myth could convince us that the primordial dangers of desire could be avoided through "mature genital sex"? But sex always draws on the primitive realm of childhood body experience. It isn't just victims of trauma, abuse, or incest who are in danger here. Every human being seeking sexual gratification enters this perilous erotic zone. The childhood body is never entirely outgrown, no matter how "mature" we are. The childhood body is always present, ready to awaken, to remember, to want, to want again, to be submerged again in this oceanic pool of primal needs and cravings, frustrations, and fulfillments.

No wonder we are afraid. If we look at the fears unleashed by our sexual remembering of the childhood body, we will find, as many women have, an entire catalog of potential dangers:

1. the vulnerability that arises from the naked sensitivity and innocence of a defenseless baby

2. the adult sense of childish "silliness" when we return to the childhood body and engage in "regressive" body explorations

3. an ideological judgment about politically correct behavior

4. the danger that unconscious childhood memories are called up, triggering conflict with our adult self-image or the story we have told ourselves about our childhood

5. our unusually high demands for something very particular, the nonfulfillment of which leads to primal frustration and rage

6. the danger that any expression of such wishes and demands implies a criticism of our lover, who hasn't figured them out yet, who will have to be taught to know and fulfill them, and who may not be capable of doing so

7. fear that the satisfaction of such strong needs could be withheld once they are made known, and that this knowledge can be used to humiliate and ridicule us

8. the possibility that reliving the neediness of infancy can

bring up a feeling of desperate dependency and threaten our sense of established power

9.   the danger that one could be turned into a sexual slave because the pleasure of fulfilled wishes is so intense and acute

Petra liked spelling out this catalog of potential dangers in our sessions. With every new listing, she felt relieved of shame and guilt. If this was everybody's problem, not just her incapacity, her inhibition, then perhaps there was hope. If it wasn't her fault and not Selena's either, then she could admit her shameful, deepest longing: The need to be handled and held like an infant, suckling at the breast — while Selena, the Great Mother, the Goddess, was gently and then a little less gently touching her genitally. The mutual acceptance of this position — the infant at the Goddess' breast — provided the magical comfort and safety for Petra to go into a state of wakefully giving herself over to her lover's touch.

The revelation taught all of us a great deal. The usual psychological attitude instructs us in the incompatibility of infantile wishes and adult sexual arousal. Along with perversions, fetishes, and other disguised symbolic expressions, infantile longings are considered regressions that prevent "mature sexuality" (sic) from taking place. Especially in Petra's case, a more traditional analyst could have made the mistake of encouraging her to abandon some of these "regressive" sensual leanings. What we learned was that the opposite approach held the key to her liberation. That key was the courage to immerse herself without any barrier in the infantile body experience; to be the infant at the breast, receiving the mother's nourishment

as a complete body experience, genitals included. It took her back to a time when there simply was no separation between sucking and sensual bodily fulfillment.

And why not? It is indeed our own fear of the power of our infantile body fantasies that has persuaded us to think of them as somehow antithetical to mature sexual arousal, unless they are disguised, enacted with a stranger, or explored under the influence of drugs or alcohol — or, in the case of many men, with a paid professional.

What may sound so simple here (like the mythical pure magic that we debunked earlier) was, of course, in the reality of Petra and Selena's bed, anything but simple. It was a slow and often frightening process, in which the moments of progress threatened to completely overwhelm Petra. Sometimes she would report the experience was too good, she didn't deserve it, she wanted to move five steps back and abandon even wanting her orgasmic pleasure. She would have fierce debates and pick fights with Selena and me in session, trying to argue against what was "simply too threatening" to her. The captain of the volleyball team now was always Selena, who was accused of being greedy, controlling, insensitive…in short, "the rapist." If Petra surrendered, she maintained, she would adopt the "feminine" passive position, and they would end up exactly where she never wanted to be, in a typical patriarchal couple that just happened to share the same sex.

The results of these fights, arguments, and defenses, however, always came down on the side of truth. The truth, it turned out, was not politically correct. It wasn't even political. The truth was that once she had tasted it, Petra could not renounce the promise of ecstasy, bliss, and physical fulfillment.

Step by step, Petra went forward — and often, after a successful progression in her transformation, she broke down in a state of surprised self-discovery, overwhelming gratitude, and simultaneous doubt that it could be maintained.

I had encountered this particular gratitude before, and have met up with it since. When one lover receives from her partner the gift of living out her secret fantasy, wish, desire — receives as a gift her own body revealed in all the innocence of its original pleasure — there's an intensification of this feeling of gratitude, which sweeps over the lovers, crashing down barriers, bringing them closer than they had ever felt before.

Selena was as overwhelmed as Petra by their discoveries, and it made her doubtful about the quality of her own sexual experience.

"I can hardly believe it," she confesses one day just before our session ends, "that somebody, my dear loved one, could have an orgasm that is so totally different from mine. It could not be any more different. If I didn't know her so well I would say she swoons into it, she doesn't get excited like I do, she melts, slowly melts like butter, her breathing simply gets deeper, she sighs a bit, but not that much, and this incredible smile starts spreading all over her face, no, really, all over her body. I am in a swoon myself just watching it and being part of it. It's so gentle, like lying back on a wave that carries you safely to shore."

She pauses. Both of them glow. Petra squeezes her hand. Selena suddenly looks tearful.

"My own orgasms now seem brutal, ordinary, I don't know, they're too fast, they're no good, I'm almost ashamed of them now. I don't want them any more. I want Petra's."

Petra shouts out: "Merging, merging. See, she's at it again.... And it was all supposed to be my fault. Wasn't it?"

I say, "Maybe Selena has a secret too?"

Selena becomes teary for the first time in our work together.

"I think I feel I have been left out all this time, somehow," she confesses. "It has been all about Petra. The adult part of me is so happy about it, but another part is sad sometimes. Maybe I am still just looking at the cake with the icing, but I have not found out how to get it for myself...."

We decide that our next sessions will focus on Selena.

Selena's Secret

Of course Selena has a secret; we all do. Selena, we now find out, is not keen on letting Petra excite her and bring her to orgasm through a slow, sensual, subtle exploration of her body. In fact, the slowness and gentleness turn her off. What she wants from Petra is what Petra experienced with the dangerous captain of her high school volleyball team — rough and tumble; impetuous desire; stormy, other-possessing sex. She likes to flare up quickly, come quickly, and be done. These two women, who seemed so merged, who appeared to have been so much alike in taking pleasure in each other's soothing touch, are in fact very different. Selena likes to enter and participate in Petra's blissful state of a cuddled child, and she even finds this

oceanic, spaced-out revery of lovemaking a turn-on. But whatever Petra does for her isn't the chili stuff, the stuff she really wants. She simply is not like Petra in this, although she admires, even envies, Petra's capacity for infantile body bliss. Petra's touching of Selena over the years has not taught her anything new about the ways in which her woman-body gets excited. She has also not learned this in any of her earlier relationships, because sex had seemed so straightforward, easy, and frankly genital. It was intense and passionate for a while, it cooled down, and the couple broke up and went on to new relationships.

And so there we are. We are stuck. Petra can have orgasms with Selena. Selena can have orgasms by herself. She can even have orgasms with Petra, but she can't get excited by it. And Petra, for her part, doesn't much like the role of the impetuous captain of the volleyball team — the rapist, as she calls her. What to do?

The breakthrough comes through an unexpected fit of jealousy.

Petra reports: "There we were at the Montclair Women's Art and Culture Club, with Lakeisha and her lover. I suddenly notice that Selena pays no attention to the singer, she stares at Lakeisha as if she's hypnotized. Even after I nudge her she keeps staring. What is she staring at? Why is she staring at Lakeisha? She's known her for years. You won't believe this. I couldn't believe it. Lakeisha has her arms up, waving along with the music, and Selena is staring at Lakeisha's armpit. I would swear she even tried to sneak closer to Lakeisha, like sticking her nose in … like sniffing her out."

"Stop it, hon," Selena nudges her. "You really exaggerate," but she's laughing and blushing.

Petra doesn't miss a beat. "Exaggerating? Who was exaggerating? I know you. It made me so...so hot...with anger."

"Hot with anger?" Her formulation makes me curious. "This was a turn-on?"

The two of them stare at me, then at each other. They seem to be at a loss.

"What were you looking at, Selena?" I ask.

"Damn. I don't know. I have a thing for armpits, I guess. I guess I do. I mean, this beautiful brown skin, lighter under the arm, like a valley, suddenly opening up when the arm is raised, with its little bit of vegetation. I don't know. The curves. I mean, it just makes you want to go and graze...."

"O how poetic," Petra snorts. "I never noticed you staring at my vegetation for hours. I find this really offensive. So it's somebody else who turns you on. Now you'll end up wanting Lakeisha, not me. And for sure she'll be a great team captain for you."

I let them fight for awhile. Selena denies that she's been staring for hours, she shouts back that Petra is unfair and simply jealous, she admits that she took a peek or two, she doesn't know why, it didn't mean anything, she says she does stare at Petra's armpits, but Petra never seems to notice when she does and why would Petra notice, for that matter? It doesn't mean anything, it just doesn't, she insists.

Petra jams her fists into her hips. She becomes visibly taller and says, with an uncharacteristic, assertive tone: "Show me your armpits."

It suddenly strikes me that Selena is always dressed in tank tops. She throws up her arms. Petra stares at her. Selena takes a deep breath and closes her eyes, as if this is too much for

her. Then, she arches her back, her breasts rise, and an expression of extraordinary relief spreads across her face. Her whole body relaxes and yields itself.

"O boy," Petra says.

"There," Selena says, opening her eyes just enough. She lowers her arms and crosses them over her breasts, embracing her own shoulders. She takes another deep breath. "Now I guess you know."

"I know, I know? What do I know? What am I supposed to do now?" Petra tries to hold back a little grin that gives her away.

I say, "I had the impression you knew very well what to do when you were staring at Selena and saying 'O boy.'"

Selena chuckles. "Petra saying 'O boy'.... Not exactly PC, is it? I love it. Just go ahead, honey, we've figured it out."

Selena's armpit was the gateway, her "Open, Sesame!" All Petra had to do was pounce on it with kisses and bites to send Selena into high sexual arousal. Petra, who got creatively inspired by the discovery, invented a game she called "truffle hunt." She got a kick out of playing the role of a wild pig rummaging about in the underbrush, eager to dig up what was hidden there. This fantasy imagery allowed her to uncover a more naughty side of herself and find it a turn-on. Once she overcame the fear of being a "rapist" and, instead, became "Captain Pig," she was able to launch into the playful expression of what she previously would have called "greedy sex."

Unshaming the Body

We may wonder why Selena didn't know this secret site of her desire; why she, so well versed in the ABC of caressing, had not recognized the intimate erotic power of the armpit.

Selena began to answer this question. How could the armpit be a legitimate erotic zone when even in our everyday language, "the pits" means the most despicable, the least desirable? Women all over the Western world are constantly reminded to hide, cover up, shave, wash, perfume, cover in deodorant — in short, eliminate their armpits from view, from knowledge, from sensual discovery as an erotic zone — perhaps because there is a faint allusion to the genitals, a hidden place that is only seen when you spread a limb and reveal hair? Selena, of course, had not felt the least bit ashamed of her armpits. She didn't shave, didn't douse herself in deodorants, and wore revealing tank tops most of the time. Nevertheless, this "natural attitude" had not allowed her to break through an unconscious barrier of shame and become aware of her armpit as an essential place of desire.

Breast hair, thick eyebrows, facial hair, double chin, love handles, hairy legs, hairy belly, cellulite — these are some of the more obvious attributes women are supposed to be ashamed of, and the list could easily fill an entire page. Indeed, it could grow so long and become so detailed, we would soon arrive at the awareness that no part of a woman's body is exempt from the potential of arousing shame.

In my own language, German, this attitude towards a woman's body is openly expressed. The German word for a woman's genitals is *Scham*, literally, "shame." This is not slang, not any

kind of colloquialism. It is the standard, proper, ordinary German term. Similarly, a woman's labia are *Schamlippen*, "shame-lips." Her *mons veneris* is *Schamhügel*, "shame-hill." And her nipples, to introduce some variety, carry the appetizing name *Brustwarzen*, "breast warts."

For most of us, in most cultures, the female body is a place of shameful embarrassment, and this is true whether or not the language a woman speaks expresses this explicitly. No wonder that even a woman as experienced as Selena could spend a lifetime without having crossed the barrier of shame to discover the secret place of her most intense erotic arousal.

Selena, Petra, and I now made some interesting discoveries and together began to speculate about the experience and impact of shame. We made another catalogue to show how our society would categorize Petra and Selena's sexual experience:

- there is no sexuality at all, there is only regressive body behavior

- genital maturity has not been reached

- Petra's oceanic orgasms, with their central clitoral engagement, are a clear indication of her inability to seek, desire, or achieve mature vaginal fulfillment

- Selena's wish to have Petra linger over her armpits is an avoidance of the experience of mature breast arousal

- the fact that Selena experiences a sensation or fantasy of penetration through her lover's kissing and biting of her armpit represents an almost fetishistic insistence that her female lover indeed has a penis

ও the fact that these two women can be aroused so enthusi-
astically in these ways is a sign of their obsessive attachment
to perverse infantile behavior

ও in short, these gals are the perverse, polymorphous anti-
heroines of Freud's famous treatise on sexuality

When we composed and contemplated this ironic catalogue
of taboos, we had a long laugh; indeed, we enjoyed many
hilarious moments of quoting and dispatching authorities on
women's bodies and pleasures. We agreed that it was virtu-
ally a miracle that any woman actually knew her body and
its subjective geography.

Most of the couples I have worked with, most of the women
I have talked to, most of my own friends and past lovers
have revealed one shameful body secret or another. To my
initial surprise, all of the shameful sites contained intense
erotic potential.

We could fill half a book with the hidden secrets of feet and
toes, elbows and knees, the fold of skin behind the ear; the
pleasures to be gleaned from licking the eye, biting and chew-
ing at the hip bone, fingers tickling up the nose — all innocent
on the face of it, and all shameful when it comes to telling a
lover that this is what one likes best, perhaps even needs most,
to be truly turned on. Selena had an entire collection of "innocent" body pleasures, and yet not a single one really turned
her on except that armpit.

One woman who confided in me had always thought that
her wish for anal pleasure was a filthy, disgusting desire. What
she hated most about her body was the tingling sensation "down
there" in that hidden place. All she had found to do with it was

dream, and fantasize about some stranger she'd meet someday at her local bar.

For this woman, finding a committed lover eager to explore her body was a shock at first. With reassurance came tentative permission to explore further. Finally, after a few years, this led to the mind-blowing experience of anal orgasm, which at first she kept insisting could not possibly exist, even though she was experiencing it.

There is, of course, a place in our culture where shameful sexual truths have permission to be told and acted out. It is found wherever erotic strangers are found, in sex clubs, on street corners, in public bathrooms, in peep shows, in the elaborately staged fantasy-rooms of today's bordellos, in pornographic magazines, in the chat rooms of the Internet.

How interesting.

How is it that, conventionally, this remarkable treasure is exchanged for money rather than for love? But we know the answer to this question. Whenever you pay, you are in control, and the risk of losing yourself is kept at bay. When you've had enough, you pay and leave. When you are in danger, you don't come back. By definition, you are always with someone in a subordinate position, who is there to do your bidding and is paid not to make judgments about what that bidding is. You can reveal yourself in all your glorious shame without any real risk of being recognized.

Women don't traditionally visit prostitutes, but they do share the general culture's fascination with the erotic stranger. How is it that, even for women, this storehouse of sexual secrets is more easily exchanged with a stranger than with one's most intimate sexual partner?

We know the answer to this, too.

Revealing embarrassing truths to a stranger entails small risk, because you may never see her again. She doesn't know who you are and therefore can't judge whether your revelations are in sharp contrast to the way you normally present yourself. The two of you are very likely entering a fantasy realm where it is easy to change identities and leave behind everything that normally constitutes your life. You have no responsibility for the future of the stranger or the relationship, therefore you are unbound in your self-expression.

How very interesting.

These private, sensual, erotic longings tend to be enacted with strangers but kept out of intimate, trusting, loving, long-term relationships, where they could be invited, cultivated, even celebrated for their capacity to create intimacy and save the relationship from erotic boredom.

An Erotic Practice

The approach we have been studying in *True Secrets of Lesbian Desire* is inherently a woman's approach. Women are particularly gifted at making truth relational, making the revelation of secrets interactive, making self-knowledge of one's body dependent upon one's comfort and safety in communication with another person. To achieve this goal requires us to pass through a prolonged period of not-knowing, as we learn

together what the culture has forbidden us to know: Ourselves and our pleasure, our shame-bodies as our bodies of pleasure.

Just as couples have to find their own pet name for Love's Learning Place, we are greatly advantaged if we find a tender, funny, silly, inspiring label for the strategy that will allow us to unearth each other's secrets. In Petra's "truffle hunt," the lover's body becomes a delicious forest filled with undercover growth and hiding places. Another couple had a bent for African animals, sending out antelopes, gazelles, and long-fingered giraffes to graze and forage across their grasslands. A friend of mine found that her totem animal was the elephant, and she was surprised to see her own mouth develop into an extraordinary agile, knowing trunk. Another friend invented "the little submarine," a technique consisting of sputtering air like little exploding bubbles through her lips. When she dived to a particularly sensitive place on her lover's body, it turned out that the little submarine encountered explosive response and was able to generate unsuspected orgasmic marvels.

Sometimes the shameful secret is hidden in a fantasy. A client of mine, an avant-garde poet who despised pop writing — in particular slasher and vampire materials — found it hard to believe that her lover playfully biting the hollow behind her knee could unleash a delirium that developed into an elaborate sexual vampire game between them.

The shame-liberated, subjective body is resurrected by every woman in her own way. We can find pathways to the unknown continent of our bodies by noticing and paying attention to what turns us on and what doesn't. "Fantasy-confessionals" between lovers can be experiences of both enlightenment and

excitement. Short fantasies can tell long stories about where we come from, sexually speaking, and where we long to go.

Another good technique for overcoming the fear of shameful revelation is the practice of retiring to a safe place, like the bed, and doing what some couples call "murmuring." Murmuring could be translated as speaking below the voice; as saying what can't be said, or should not be said, but can only be whispered into the lover's ear. With that label handy, both partners know that when one of them expresses the need for murmuring, something weighs on that partner's soul and wants to be told. It could be a secret, it could be a shameful longing, it could be a hurt. Knowing a name for the process facilitates the task. Knowing a particularly appealing, funny, or tender name for it takes away half the fear of undertaking it in the first place.

Fantasy confessionals and murmuring practices belong to a larger group of strategies that many women call rituals. By the term *ritual* they mean a place and a process that can be visited and revisited at regular or irregular intervals. They mean a place that exists only between them, a place they have created by giving form to a soul desire. They mean a process that follows some simple, meaningful rules. You light a candle, burn incense, put on a favorite piece of music in order to call up the spirits that are needed in order to accomplish a difficult task. You want to invite protection when you take a risk. One couple I know goes on a particular walk to sit by a pond in a beautiful, small wood. They pick up pebbles on the way to the pond, speak their fears and their wishes, and with every one of them they launch a pebble into the lake.

"The water takes care of it," they told me. "It takes our wishes

to the ocean and back into the sky where they become rain. Every time we throw one of them we say, 'May it be,' in chorus. And we feel, this way, it will be done, it will come true. And you know what? It does."

Other women I know perform fear rituals. They write what they are most afraid of on little bits of paper, speak them aloud to one another, then burn them in the flame of a particular candle set up for the purpose.

These are only a few examples of techniques or practices that make it easier to speak the truth straight from the heart. What they all have in common is the tendency to bring the couple into a confessional closeness that leads directly into lovemaking, sometimes even in the woods. It is a breathtaking, risk-filled intimacy, in which truth-making and lovemaking and hot sex and intimate passion become one.

This need no longer sound like a paradox. Yes, our culture tells us repeatedly, in every possible way, exactly the opposite: Hot, rich, fulfilling sex is transient; it belongs to the passionate beginning of a relationship, or to an encounter between strangers; it thrives on distance, estrangement, fights; it needs violence, as we have already described in detail. But we have now discovered that trust and safety are preconditions for lasting, passionate intimacy. In a long-term relationship, the quality of truth can be worked out and refined. More than likely, this rare truth doesn't initially know or discover itself until a relationship has matured and helped both partners to overcome their culturally and socially conditioned shame.

What?

A sexuality we scarcely dare imagine?

Ripened between two people who have known each other

long enough to take ultimate risks?

The sexuality for which we ardently long, waiting for us in the very bed we thought had condemned it to death?

You bet!

Books Mentioned in the Text

Allison, Dorothy. "Public Silence, Private Terror." In *Skin: Talking about Sex, Class & Literature*. Ithaca: Firebrand Books,1994: 112.

Bohan, Janis S., and Glenda M. Russell, eds. *Conversations about Psychology and Sexual Orientation*. New York: New York University Press, 1999. This book provides a vast reading list on sex therapy and clinical therapy issues for women.

Freud, Sigmund. *Three Essays on the Theory of Sexuality*. New York: Basic Books, 1988.

Iasenza, Suzanne. "The Big Lie: Debunking Lesbian Bed Death." *In the Family, the Magazine for Lesbians, Gays, Bisexuals and their Relations* (April 1999): 8.

Lorde, Audre. *Sister Outsider*. Freedom, CA: The Crossing Press, 1984: 10, 128.

Minkowitz, Donna. *Ferocious Romance: What My Encounters with the Right Taught Me about Sex, God, and Fury*. New York: The Free Press, 1998.

Reich, Wilhelm. *The Function of the Orgasm: Sex-Economic Problems of Biological Energy*. New York: Noonday Press, 1986.

Rich, Adrienne. *On Lies, Secrets, and Silence: Selected Prose 1966-1978*. New York: Norton & Co, 1979: 188.

—. Introduction to "Compulsory Heterosexuality and Lesbian Existence." *Sign* V (summer 1980).

Steinem, Gloria. "Ms.behavin' Again," interview by Claudia Dreifus, *Modern Maturity* (May-June 1999): 53.

Wolf, Naomi. *Promiscuities: The Secret Struggle for Womanhood*. New York: Fawcett Columbine,1997:181.This book has an excellent reading list.

⧠ A book not mentioned, but a source of great inspiration and courage in my thinking about truth-telling is Michelle Citron's *Home Movies and Other Necessary Fictions*, Minneapolis, University of Minnesota Press, 1999.